SECRETS TO YOUTHFUL AGING

Leo F. Semacio
Secrets to Youthful Aging

Published by Spines
ISBN: 979-8-89383-312-6

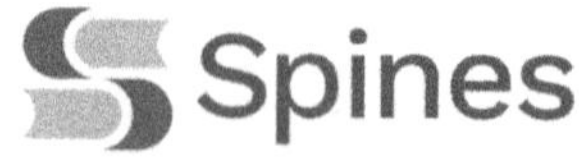

SECRETS TO YOUTHFUL AGING

(STRATEGIES REVEALED)

LEO F. SEMACIO

DEDICATION

To The Very Young

Generation Alpha (2015 - -)

Generation Z (1996 – 2015)

To today's vibrant and aspiring youth, this book is a heartfelt dedication to the invaluable treasure trove of old age. As you stand on the precipice of your journey through life, it's essential to recognize and honor the profound wisdom, resilience, and beauty that characterize the later years of your life. Old age is not merely a destination but a culmination of experiences, a reservoir of knowledge and wisdom waiting for you to tap.

You are like the fresh green leaves of spring, swaying in the cold wind of late winter, its sprig ready to bear fruit for summer's bloom and the goodness of harvest in autumn.

The Art of Gratitude

As you forge ahead, it's crucial to recognize the art of gratitude emanating from older adults' hearts. Gratitude for the simple joys, enduring relationships, and precious moments constitute a well-lived life. Your gratitude is a gentle reminder to cherish the present, savor the journey, and acknowledge the beauty of every fleeting moment you may have while trudging for dear life. Life is meant to be lived; it is intended to be well-lived.

A Fountain of Stories

Old age is a fountain of stories, each uniquely blending love, loss, triumph, laughter, tears, and sorrows. Our tales are anecdotes and lessons encapsulated in our own narratives. Listening to our stories is an opportunity to glean insights, perspectives, and timeless truths that transcend the boundaries of time.

Guides on the Path of Compassion

Older adults are your guides on the path of compassion. Our presence teaches you the significance of empathy, kindness, and understanding. As you embark on your journey, remember that embracing the wisdom of older adults is an act of compassion, a way of acknowledging the shared humanity that unites us all.

Conclusion

To the very young and vibrant, let this be a dedication to you—a tribute to the living reservoirs of wisdom, resilience, and stories. As you carve your own path, may you recognize the importance of standing on the shoulders of those who have tread before you. In the embrace of old age, discover the timeless truths that connect generations. Let the wisdom of ages guide you on your journey of growth, compassion, and fulfillment.

To The Not-So-Young

Millennials (1981 – 1995)

Generation X (1965 – 1980)

This book is a heartfelt dedication to you—the not-so-young ones, those who have traversed the varied landscapes of life and now stand at the threshold of the golden years. As life's pace may seem slow, it's crucial to acknowledge the profound value and richness of experience that define this chapter of your life. To those who carry the weight of years with grace, this is a tribute to the wisdom, resilience, strength, and enduring spirit accompanying the journey into old age.

The Tapestry of Experience

You, the not-so-young individuals, are akin to master weavers. You have crafted the tapestry of your lives with threads of joy, sorrow, love, and perseverance. Each strand you weave is a testament to the myriad experiences that have shaped you into who you are today. The richness of this tapestry imparts a unique and irreplaceable beauty to the fabric of your existence, a masterpiece of a lifetime.

A Symphony of Relationships

You, the not-so-young, have conducted the symphony of relationships, weaving a complex but harmonious melody with members of your family, friends, and society. Your relationships carry the weight of shared history, echoing the laughter, tears, and shared moments that form the foundation of meaningful connections.

The Art of Adaptation

The age of the not-so-young is a testament to the art of adaptation. You, the not-so-young, have displayed remarkable adaptability. Whether navigating career changes, weathering personal storms, or embracing the inevitability of physical changes, you embody the strength of adapting to life's ever-changing landscape.

Cultivators of Patience

You, the not-so-young, are cultivators of patience, having weathered the storms of impatience and haste that characterize the earlier years. With time, you have learned to appreciate the beauty of patience, understanding that some things are worth waiting for and that life unfolds at its own pace.

Keepers of Stories

In your not-so-young years, you become keepers of stories—chroniclers of a lifetime's worth of experiences. The stories you share are not just personal narratives but a collective wisdom that spans generations. Listening to these stories is an opportunity to gain insights, learn from history, and appreciate the resilience that has sustained you through the test of time.

Masters of Gratitude

You, the not-so-young, are masters of gratitude, appreciating life's simplicity. Gratitude becomes a lens through which you view the world, recognizing the blessings in each moment, the beauty in small gestures, and the value of a life well lived with purpose and intention.

Conclusion

To you, the not-so-young, this book is a dedication to your wisdom, resilience, and the profound value you bring to the tapestry of human existence. Embrace the richness of your experiences, for you are the jewels that adorn the fabric of your life. As you continue your journey into the golden years, may you find fulfillment in the depth of your connections, the wisdom you share, and the enduring spirit that defines this remarkable chapter of your life.

To The Once-Upon-A-Time Young

Baby Boomers (1946 – 1964)

Silent Generation (1928 – 1945)

Greatest Generation (1901 – 1927)

This book is a contemplative message addressing the inevitability of old age to the once-upon-a-time young, whose days were adorned with the hues of dreams and the promise of endless possibilities. As we reflect on the passage of time and the transformation of our narrative, let these words serve as a companion on the journey into the golden years. This journey is about self-discovery and embracing the profound beauty of growing old.

The Tapestry of Youth

We, the once-upon-a-time young, wove the tapestry of our youth with the threads of curiosity, boundless energy, and the thrill of the unknown. Each day was an adventure, and the future beckoned with the allure of uncharted territories. Our dreams were the compass guiding our endeavors, and the world was a canvas awaiting the brushstrokes of our ambitions.

Navigating the Rapids of Change

Time is a relentless river; as the currents carried us forward, we faced the rapids of change. Life's unpredictable twists and turns may have shaped us in ways you couldn't foresee. Through career shifts, personal challenges, and the ebb and flow of relationships, we learned to navigate the waters with resilience and strength, adapting to the evolving landscapes of our own story.

The Legacy of Relationships

In the days of once upon a time, relationships were a kaleidoscope of emotions—love, friendship, heartbreak, and joy. As the years unfolded, the relationships we nurtured became a significant part of our legacy. The bonds we forged with family, friends, and those who touched our hearts and even those we felt carried the weight of shared experiences, forming the foundation of a life well-lived.

Wisdom Woven by Time

Old age is not merely the twilight of life but the culmination of a journey etched with experiences, lessons, and self-discovery. Each wrinkle on our faces tells a story, and each gray hair is a badge of honor, signifying the wisdom woven by the hands of time. As we embrace the not-so-young years, let the depth of our insights become a guiding light for those who follow in our footsteps.

Embracing the Beauty of Impermanence

We, the once upon a time young, are often enamored with permanence. Yet, the wisdom that old age imparts lies in recognizing the beauty of impermanence. Life is a transient dance, and every step is a fleeting moment of change embodied in the priceless memories we left behind. Embrace the present, savor the past, accept the future, and find solace in the understanding that change is the only constant event in our lifetime.

Cultivating Gratitude

In our younger days, it was easy to overlook the simple joys amidst the clamor of ambitions. Old age invites us to cultivate gratitude, a practice that transforms ordinary moments into extraordinary blessings. We find gratitude in the warmness of the sun, the banter of our dearly beloved, and the quiet beauty of a life well-lived.

Conclusion

To the once-upon-a-time young, as we stand on the threshold of the golden years and the twilight of our lives, remember that aging is not a fading away but a blossoming phase of our life into a new season of tomorrow. Embrace the wrinkles as etchings of laughter, cherish the gray hairs as silver crowns of wisdom, and let the journey into old age continue the epic tale we started once upon a time. May the chapters ahead be filled with the resonance of a rich life, maybe not materially, but beyond material things, and may we discover the profound beauty that comes beyond while growing old.

DISCLOSURE STATEMENT

The information provided herein is not intended as medical advice. It is based solely on personal experience and should not be construed as a substitute for professional medical advice, diagnosis, or treatment. Always seek the advice of your physician or other qualified health provider with any questions you may have regarding a medical condition. Reliance on any information provided here is solely at your own risk.

CONTENTS

PREFACE

This preface invites you to traverse the landscapes of time and experiences as you explore aging. The journey into the world of aging is not merely a chronological progression but a multidimensional odyssey that unfolds in the intricate tapestry of life. The following pages explore the complexities, nuances, and profound beauty of the aging process. Join me in exploring the secrets of the mythical and fabled "fountain of youth," which may be accessible at hand.

The notion of aging has evolved beyond mere clock ticking or the tallying of years. It is an experiential journey, a continuum marked by the indelible imprints of joy, challenges, wisdom, and resilience. This preface sets the stage for exploring the multifaceted aspects of aging, seeking to unveil the layers that define this transformative passage of time and into aging.

Aging is not a singular narrative but a mosaic of stories uniquely painted by the strokes of individual experiences. In this book, we aim to celebrate the richness of these stories—the laughter, the tears, the triumphs, the heartaches, and the reflections that characterize the journey into the later years. It is an acknowledgment that every individual's path through aging is distinctive and shaped by many societal influences and personal choices.

Furthermore, this preface sets the tone for a nuanced understanding of aging that transcends stereotypes and embraces the diversity within the aging population. Dispelling myths, challenging preconceptions, and acknowledging the tenacity and vibrancy that often characterize older individuals are the central themes that guide our very own personal narrative.

In the following pages, we will explore various facets of aging, including physical health, mental well-being, social connections, and the intersection of aging with broader societal themes. We will navigate the terrain of ageism, celebrating the strengths of older individuals while recognizing the challenges we may face in life. The importance of intergenerational connections, the role of community, and evolving perspectives on what it means to age gracefully will be an integral part of why I wrote this book.

As we embark on this journey, I desire readers to find inspiration, insights, and a deeper appreciation for the profound beauty that accompanies the process of aging. Through the words that unfold in the subsequent chapters, I invite you to engage in a reflective dialogue about our journey, to share in the collective wisdom of those who have traversed the path before us, and to embrace the aging process with a spirit of curiosity and celebration, thankful that our Creator had given us the chance and opportunity to experience the marvels of life, especially in the process of aging.

May this book serve as a companion, a guide, and a source of inspiration for all who embark on the journey of aging —whether in the bloom of youth, the prime of life, or the embrace of later years. Together, let us explore the ever-evolving landscapes of aging, recognizing it not as a destination but as an ongoing, transformative odyssey that enriches the very fabric of our existence – until the twilight moment of our lifetime.

INTRODUCTION
AGING? ANYONE?

We panic when we see a strand of grey hair on our forehead, cringe when we hear our knees cracking, complain about waking up in the middle of the night and finding it hard to sleep again, and ask ourselves, "Are these the signs of old age?"

As we settle down to try to grasp reality versus ethereal thinking, we try to justify that there is nothing to worry about. Instead, it is something we should be proud of and happy about. We have reached a stage of life that some were not privileged to experience.

We evaluate and calculate that aging is the number of years we have lived. Still, we are also confronted with the reality that this is not the case. We know of someone who is 55 years old but looks more youthful and healthier than the other guy who is 35 years old but looks aged and sickly. Why is this so? It is better to delve into a careful or detailed study of information on what causes aging and premature aging.

As we all know, aging is a natural and inevitable process that all living organisms, including you and me, should undergo throughout our lives. The process is caused by the power and effect or the combination of any or all factors, e.g., genetic, environmental, lifestyle, etc.

Universally, aging is a process that exempts no one. However, the effects and degree of aging vary to a great degree and extent among individuals. As living creatures, we are subjected to a gradual decline in the efficacy of our bodies' biological processes. Over a period of time, cells divide, and the telomeres of our chromosomes tend to shorten, leading to cellular senescence or cell death. As a result, the process gives way to the aging of our tissues and organs. This causes our skin to reduce elasticity, decrease muscle mass, and alter cognitive performance. This must be why, as we age, we seem to shrink in size and become recognizably old, even looking into our own silhouette.

Aging is also genetically influenced. Some individuals may inherit genes that are resilient to certain age-related situations, while others may have a genetic inclination to age-related illnesses. Aging is a complicated and multifaceted process that our physical body undergoes.

Factors like genetics, environment, and lifestyle influence it. Although the mechanism of our body's aging process is not fully understood, several scientific principles have tried to explain the causes of aging.

No one is exempt from aging—that is a brutal fact—but premature aging happens faster than it should to some unlucky souls. Signs of early aging usually appear in our skin. The most common symptoms are wrinkles, age spots, sagging, dryness, loss of skin tone, and hair growing white or gray. In some cases, the hairline expands in the forehead, and temples widen, with hair thinning at the top of the head, and some end up without hair at all.

Genetics is only one element of the mystery of aging. Other factors, like diet, exercise, stress, exposure to hazardous elements, etc., are also involved. In the later part of this book, we will discuss the causes of aging that play crucial roles in an individual's aging.

Being at risk for various health conditions is also considered to cause aging. The tendency of our immune system to weaken with age is also the cause of susceptibility to infections and other ailments in elderlies. With all of these challenges, it is good to note that advancements in healthcare and lifestyle interference may impact the process of aging and alleviate its causes. In addition, ongoing research on the biology of aging may uncover new methods to slow down or even reverse certain aspects of the aging process.

It is important to note that aging is a natural and normal phenomenon of humankind's life cycle and that stakeholders should accept it with a positive mindset. Several older adults go on with life, living an active, fulfilling life and enjoying a prosperous social community relationship. Moreover, communities worldwide are accepting the demographic of an aging population. They are looking for ways to give support and resources to older members of society to maintain a high quality of life as they age.

To conclude, the complexity of the aging process brings challenges and changes that can lead to opportunities for an individual to age gracefully by adopting healthy habits and engaging in meaningful activities. Fully understanding and directing efforts to several factors associated with aging contributes to a more comprehensive and optimistic viewpoint on this natural phase of life no one is exempt from passing through.

To some, these symptoms are alarming, and they consciously seek solutions to save themselves from the onset of premature aging or, to some extent, delay the process.

PART ONE
CAUSES OF AGING

Understanding the causes of aging on a personal basis can have implications in our day-to-day lives. Knowing the causes of aging can empower us to influence our approaches to health and well-being positively. Being aware of its causes makes us conscious of the factors contributing to why and how we age. Awareness also motivates us to take preventative measures against age-related diseases. We will then understand how all the risk factors for age-related conditions, e.g., genetic and environmental, may benefit from tailored medical approaches or interventions.

Furthermore, knowledge of the causes of aging can inform us when planning for our future, which may contribute to more realistic expectations about health and lifestyle in years to come. We then are empowered to take an active role in our own aging process that may lead to a proactive approach, fostering a positive mindset and willingness to adopt health habits to prevent or reverse the process of aging. We then are empowered to make informed decisions about lifestyle, nutrition, and overall health habits, resulting in a higher quality of life.

In essence, knowing the causes of aging on a personal level empowers us to make choices that can positively influence our health, well-being, and overall life satisfaction as we navigate the aging process.

Understanding the causes of aging is a crucial area of scientific research with broad implications for various fields, including medicine, biology, and public health. By understanding the mystery of aging, researchers can find ways to develop interventions and therapies to help slow down or potentially reverse the aging process. This could lead to the development of treatments for age-related ailments and health-related conditions. Identifying the causes of aging may contribute to increasing the human lifespan and improving the quality of life in our old age. But it does not stop from there; investigating the causes of aging is about enhancing general health and well-being as we go through the process of aging.

CHAPTER 1
STRESS

I put stress as Number 1 on the list because I consider this factor very significant in causing one to age. I cannot emphasize much of its importance in considering stress as the number one factor in premature aging. I know many of our friends and relatives who are stressed about innuendos in life; lo and behold, they look old for their age. It is a fact that in our day-to-day living, we are highly exposed to and bombarded with various stressful elements like physical, emotional, psychological, financial, relational, environmental, etc., you name it, you got it.

Stress, especially chronic or prolonged, can contribute to the aging process through our body's various physiological and psychological mechanisms. Stress is a complex physiological response that can impact various systems in the body, and chronic stress has been associated with the aging process. The relationship between stress and aging is symbiotic and multifaceted, involving biological, psychological, and behavioral factors that can impact the body and contribute to premature aging.

Clinically, stress can cause hair loss and high blood pressure and make our body insulin-resistant. So, stressing out about a given situation in our life will only worsen it. I don't understand why we love to stress out and dwell on a given stressful situation. We love to wallow, dwell on it, and savor the bitterness of the sad and stressful situation. Sad as it is. We love drama in real life.

Here are some key types of stress that may influence aging:

Financial Stress

Financial stress, or the strain associated with economic concerns and financial instability, can contribute to the aging process through various physiological and psychological pathways. While financial stress does not directly cause aging, the associated factors and responses to stress negatively affect our overall well-being, especially our health, potentially accelerating the aging process.

Here are some ways in which financial stress may impact aging:

Chronic Stress Response

Persistent financial stress can lead to chronic activation of the body's stress response system, resulting in a prolonged elevation of the cortisol stress hormone, known to cause health issues like cardiovascular problems, impaired immune system, and inflammation, factors linked to aging resulting in prolonged elevation.

Mental Health Impact

Financial stress is often linked to mental health issues such as anxiety and depression, which, when chronic, can give in to cognitive decline with the increased risk of neurodegenerative disorders, potentially accelerating the aging of the brain. The sufferer tends to become forgetful, jittery, and hyper-sensitive to stressful events. Some, even when they cannot cope or when the coping mechanism cannot tolerate stress anymore, become mentally derailed, which is more depressing, especially for the family.

Health Behavior Changes

Financial stress may lead to unhealthy coping mechanisms, such as increased smoking, excessive alcohol consumption, poor dietary choices, or loss of appetite that contribute to the acceleration of the aging process. When under stress, our chest seems to tighten and feel heavy. We breathe rapidly and palpitate, and our pulse and heartbeat are accelerated, stressing the heart. Though there is no direct evidence to suggest that the acceleration of pulse and heartbeat can cause aging, the risk of having a heart disease is imminent.

Sleep Disturbances

Financial worries can cause sleep disturbances, such as insomnia or poor sleep quality. Disrupted sleep patterns are associated with various health issues, including cardiovascular problems and cognitive decline, which contribute to the aging process. Looking in the mirror, one sees dark circles paired with an unpleasant, ugly look of puffy bags around the eyes. When sleep is deprived, one does not like to see one's looks in the mirror.

Impact on Relationships

Financial stress can strain relationships, leading to conflicts. Money is a very sensitive issue, sometimes resulting in conflict and even a heated confrontation. Stress in a strained relationship has adverse effects on an individual's mental and emotional well-being and has been linked to accelerated aging.

Access to Healthcare

Financial stress may limit access to healthcare, preventing individuals from seeking timely medical attention and preventive care. Lack of healthcare can lead to the development of chronic conditions and exacerbate the aging process. Many of our friends cannot see a doctor regularly because of financial constraints. They are "forced" to go to an emergency room only when their health is in jeopardy, when they are in a serious condition, or when their situation is between life and death.

Lifestyle Changes

Financial stress may result in lifestyle changes, such as reduced physical and leisure activities. A sedentary lifestyle and lack of engagement in enjoyable activities can contribute to aging-related health issues. Financial constraints can limit the ability of older people or couples to engage in social activities or even the opportunity to travel, leading to feelings of isolation and even depression, impacting their overall relationship satisfaction.

Accelerated Cellular Aging

Financial stress, when chronic, is known to be associated with cellular aging. The length of telomeres, the protective caps at the end of our chromosomes, and changes in size are related to cellular longevity and may cause cellular aging and, eventually, premature aging.

It's essential to recognize that the relationship between financial stress and aging is complex, and every individual response may vary. Finding healthy coping mechanisms, seeking social support, and developing effective financial management strategies are crucial for mitigating the potential adverse effects of financial stress on both physical and mental health.

Physical Stress

Physical stress can contribute to the aging process through various physiological mechanisms. While some level of physical stress is a natural and necessary part of our lives, chronic or excessive physical stress can harm our bodies over time.

Here are some ways in which physical stress may contribute to aging:

Oxidative Stress

Physical stress, such as intense exercise or exposure to environmental toxins, can increase the production of free radicals in the body. This process is called oxidative stress, wherein reactive free radicals contribute to damaging cells and cause aging and various age-related diseases.

Inflammation

Intense physical stress, particularly when it leads to overtraining or repetitive strain on the body, can trigger inflammation. Chronic inflammation is linked to aging and is associated with conditions such as arthritis, cardiovascular disease, and neurodegenerative disorders.

Hormonal Changes

Prolonged physical stress can impact the balance of hormones in the body. For example, excessive exercise may lead to elevated cortisol levels, which, when chronic, can contribute to metabolic dysfunction and other factors associated with aging.

Telomere Shortening

Physical stress, especially repetitive strain or intense exercise, has been associated with accelerated telomere shortening. Telomeres are the protective cap at each chromosome and are linked to cellular aging.

Muscle and Joint Wear and Tear

The wear and tear caused by continuous physical stress without adequate recovery can result in conditions such as osteoarthritis and a decline in overall physical function, contributing to premature aging.

Immune System Suppression

Exposure to prolonged physical stress suppresses the immune system, making the body vulnerable to illnesses and infections. A weakened immune system is associated with age-related health issues.

Cardiovascular Strain

Intense physical stress, especially in individuals with pre-existing cardiovascular conditions, can place strain on the heart and blood vessels that will contribute to cardiovascular diseases associated with aging.

Sleep Disruption

Overtraining or excessive physical stress can disrupt sleep patterns. Poor sleep quality and insufficient rest can lead to metabolic dysfunction and cognitive decline, which are linked to aging.

Moderate and appropriately managed physical stress, such as regular exercise, can provide numerous health benefits and may slow aging. Therefore, it is essential to balance physical activity and rest simultaneously, avoiding excessive strain and ensuring that the body has the opportunity to recover. Listening to one's body, incorporating adequate recovery strategies, and adjusting physical activity levels based on individual fitness and health status are essential for promoting overall health and well-being.

Job-Related Stress

Job-related stress, often associated with high demands, pressure, and challenges in the workplace, can contribute to the aging process through various physical and psychological mechanisms. The impact of job-related stress on aging is complex and can manifest in several ways:

Chronic Activation of the Stress Response

Persistent job-related stress can lead to the chronic activation of the body's stress response system, in which our body releases a hormone called cortisol, which, if elevated over an extended period of time, may contribute to physiological changes associated with aging.

Inflammation

Chronic stress at work has been linked to increased inflammation, a natural immune response. However, regular, low-grade inflammation is associated with illnesses like cardiovascular and neurodegenerative disorders, which are age-related diseases.

Cardiovascular Strain

High stress levels, especially in high-pressure work environments, can contribute to cardiovascular strain. This may lead to elevated blood pressure, increased heart rate, and other cardiovascular issues associated with aging. Try to check your blood pressure after a long, tedious, stressful day at work. You will not be surprised if it is at its highest point.

Sleep Disruption

We have a favorite tendency to bring our problems from the office to home, or vice versa. We tend to think about our jobs while trying to get a good night's sleep. Worse, we even get nightmares, especially if we have some serious cases that are job-related at hand. Job-related stress can interfere with the quality and quantity of our sleep. The effect of disrupted sleep is a decline of cognitive capabilities, weakened immune systems, and an increased risk of various diseases associated with aging, known to have been linked to poor sleeping habits.

Mental Health Impact

Job-related stress can contribute to mental health issues such as anxiety and depression. These conditions are associated with cognitive decline and an increased risk of age-related neurodegenerative disorders. "My job is driving me crazy!" we used to say.

Unhealthy Coping Mechanisms

Individuals experiencing job-related stress may adopt unhealthy coping mechanisms, such as smoking, excessive alcohol consumption, or poor dietary choices, as mentioned in the previous chapter. These behaviors can contribute to aging and increase the risk of age-related diseases. This is very common for people who are stressed by their dear livelihood. This is one of the reasons why watering holes near offices proliferate profitably: we tend to get ourselves trying to relax after a hard day's work. We tend to justify that we deserve to relax a bit, but we cannot do away with smoking and drinking with a "valid" justification that we need to have a break.

Accelerated Cellular Aging

Some research suggests that chronic stress, including work-related stress, may be associated with accelerated cellular aging, as measured by changes in telomere length. Protective caps at each end of our telomeres are affiliated with our cellular longevity.

Reduced Function of the Immune System

Prolonged stress reduces the practical function of the immune system in every individual, making them susceptible to infections and various diseases. A weakened immune system function is a factor associated with aging. Have you ever noticed that you always get sick if you are stressed, especially at work? And we always say, "This job is killing me?"

Poor Work-Life Balance

Imbalances between work and personal life can contribute to stress. Chronic overwork and lack of time for relaxation and personal pursuits can negatively affect overall well-being and accelerate aging.

It's important to note that individuals respond differently to job-related stress, and the impact on aging can vary. Implementing effective stress management techniques, promoting a healthy work-life balance, and seeking social support can help alleviate the adverse effects of job-related stress on physical and mental health. Creating a supportive work environment and addressing systemic factors contributing to stress can also benefit employee's well-being. It is a good idea to join any group or community that will divert your stress to the community's stress-relieving activities. We have a lot of community groups that we can join, depending on your interest and inclination. There are a lot of groups to join, like community service, volunteer services, social amelioration, charity work, etc. Or better yet, be involved in any hobbies that interest you, like baking, gardening, writing, singing, etc. Maybe along the way, you may make money with this side hustle or, most probably or eventually, leave your stressful job to make it a full-time business. Any bright idea?

Emotional and Psychological Stress

Emotional and psychological stress, such as chronic worry, anxiety, or depressive symptoms, can have physical effects on our bodies. We combine these two stressors into one because they involve our minds, feelings, sentiments, and passions. We classically identify this person as the "worrier" type of personality.

Emotional and psychological stress may contribute to inflammation, oxidative stress, and hormonal imbalances, all associated with accelerated aging.

Lifestyle-Related Stress

An unhealthy lifestyle, like an unhealthy diet, substance abuse, and lack of physical activities, can result in stress and accelerate aging. These factors can affect overall health and increase the risk of age-related diseases.

Note From the Author

Please note that stress affects different individuals, and its impact on aging is influenced by several factors, including overall health, genetics, and each individual's coping mechanism. When managed through healthy lifestyle approaches, relaxation techniques, social support, and mindful practices can help mitigate its adverse effects on aging and overall well-being.

It is important to note that individual responses to stress can vary, and not everyone will experience the same effects. Additionally, adopting stress management strategies, such as relaxing exercises, meditation, yoga, and social support from peers, can aid in alleviating the adverse effects of chronic stress, like premature aging. Overall, the relationship between stress and aging is an active area of research, and scientists continue to explore the intricate mechanisms involved in premature aging.

Stress, if at an elevated rate, increases the risk for several physical and mental health issues like anxiety, depression, digestive tract problems, unexplained headaches, including muscle and body pain, heart disease, heart attack, high blood pressure, stroke, sleep problems, weight gain, memory loss, and concentration impairment.

A lot of the aging symptoms can be the result of stress. The stress you get from work, co-workers, and boss is overwhelming. When you get home, you will be bombarded with stress from your own family, like marital relationship issues, sibling rivalries, problems rearing up children, financial problems, and all other sorts of mundane events in life that can lead to problems like hair loss, diabetes, high blood pressure, and other health issues. Too much stress can make your body insulin-resistant, which will result in diabetes.

According to **bld. Wealth** *stress makes you sick, and we don't need to elaborate on each cause. The following are the end-result stress causes:*

1. *Sleeping problems*
2. *Panic Attacks*
3. *Chest Pains*
4. *Muscle Tension*
5. *Upset Stomach*
6. *Acid Reflux*
7. *Lack of Focus*

8. *Hair Loss*
9. *Lethargy*
10. *Increased Heart Rate*
11. *Adrenal Fatigue*
12. *Reduced Sex Drive*

However, while it may seem like common knowledge that stress can make you sick, explaining and educating about the mechanisms and consequences of stress on health remains valuable for promoting health literacy and encouraging individuals to take proactive steps to manage stress effectively.

CHAPTER 2
LIFESTYLE

Physical activity is any movement of our skeletal muscles that needs energy to move around, to change place, position, or posture. If we exercise regularly, it will have substantial benefits on our physical and mental health. Exercise also supports cognitive function and emotional well-being, aside from helping to rejuvenate our muscle mass, bone density, and cardiovascular wellness. It also reinforces our body to lower the risk of osteoporosis and heart disease.

Thus, a non-active or sedentary way of life can accelerate our body's aging process, partnering with a very high risk of age-related health issues.

Time Magazine, in its article dated January 18, 2017, entitled "Sitting Too Much Ages You By 8 Years," disclosed that too much sitting throughout the day can cause several illnesses, including obesity, heart disease, diabetes, and even early demise.

That being said, premature aging will soon take its toll when our bodies are not in good, healthy condition. You might have a family member or a close relative or friend who, at age 35, looks like a 60-year-old senior citizen. On the contrary, we may have some co-workers, friends, or relatives who, at 70 years old, look like just a day old on their 50th birthday.

Our lifestyle has a significant effect on our body's aging process. A passive and lazy lifestyle may lead to an earlier aging of our body than usual. With the new generation and modern culture, and, of course, the advent of computers and social media, we are tempted to squander our precious time on social media. But, mind you, social media has its pros and cons. It depends on how you use it.

How we live our lives has a compelling effect on the aging process, influencing both the rate of aging and our overall well-being as we grow older. Choices of living a healthy lifestyle can contribute to positive aging, while certain behaviors may accelerate premature aging. Significantly, our lifestyle is essential to our longevity and biological aging. We will discuss all the lifestyles later in this book to understand how lifestyle affects our body's aging process.

An inactive or sedentary lifestyle can contribute to various age-related health issues. Here are some ways in which an inactive lifestyle affects aging:

Muscle Atrophy

Sarcopenia, or muscle wasting, is another term for Muscle atrophy, which refers to the gradual loss of muscle mass and strength.

It is a common phenomenon associated with aging, and its impact on an individual is significant because it affects overall health and well-being.

Several factors that contribute to muscle atrophy in the aging process are as follows:

Decreased Protein Synthesis

Aging is associated with a decline in the body's ability to synthesize proteins, including those needed for muscle maintenance and repair. Over time, this can lead to a net loss of muscle tissue.

Hormonal Changes

Changes in hormonal levels, such as a decrease in growth hormone, testosterone, and insulin-like growth factor 1 (IGF-1), can contribute to muscle atrophy. These hormones play essential roles in maintaining muscle mass and promoting protein synthesis.

Nutrient Deficiency

Inadequate intake of essential nutrients, especially protein and amino acids, can contribute to muscle atrophy. Proper nutrition is crucial for maintaining muscle mass and preventing age-related muscle loss.

Neuromuscular Changes

Changes in the nervous system are associated with aging, leading to a decline in motor neurons and neuromuscular junctions. This can reduce muscle activation and contribute to muscle wasting.

Chronic Inflammation

Chronic inflammation, a common feature of aging, can negatively impact muscle tissue. Inflammation may disrupt the balance between muscle protein synthesis and breakdown, leading to muscle loss.

The consequences of muscle atrophy in aging include:

Decreased Strength and Functionality

Muscle atrophy can lead to a decline in overall strength and physical function, making daily activities more challenging.

Increased Risk of Falls and Fractures

Weakened muscles can accelerate the dangers of falls and broken bones, resulting in severe consequences for older people.

Impaired Metabolism

Muscle tissue plays a crucial role in maintaining metabolic health. Muscle atrophy can contribute to metabolic disturbances and conditions like insulin resistance.

Loss of Independence

As muscle mass and strength decline, individuals may lose independence and rely more on assistance for daily activities.

Adopting a lifestyle that includes regular exercise, adequate nutrition, and other habits that support muscle health is essential to mitigate the effects of muscle atrophy and promote healthy aging. Resistance training, in particular, prevents and reverses muscle atrophy in older adults.

Decreased Protein Synthesis

Aging is associated with a decline in the body's ability to synthesize proteins, including those needed for muscle maintenance and repair. Over time, this can lead to a net loss of muscle tissue.

Hormonal Changes

Changes in hormonal levels, such as a decrease in growth hormone, testosterone, and insulin-like growth factor 1 (IGF-1), can contribute to muscle atrophy. These hormones play essential roles in maintaining muscle mass and promoting protein synthesis.

Nutrient Deficiency

Inadequate intake of essential nutrients, especially protein and amino acids, can contribute to muscle atrophy. Proper nutrition is crucial for maintaining muscle mass and preventing age-related muscle loss.

Neuromuscular Changes

Changes in the nervous system are associated with aging, leading to a decline in motor neurons and neuromuscular junctions. This can reduce muscle activation and contribute to muscle wasting.

Chronic Inflammation

Chronic inflammation, a common feature of aging, can negatively impact muscle tissue. Inflammation may disrupt the balance between muscle protein synthesis and breakdown, leading to muscle loss.

Adopting a lifestyle that includes regular exercise, adequate nutrition, and other habits that support muscle health is essential to mitigate the effects of muscle atrophy and promote healthy aging. Resistance training, in particular, prevents and reverses muscle atrophy in older adults.

Bone Health

Our bone needs physical activities to maintain its density and strength. Being inactive can result in the loss of bone mass, which will lead to conditions like osteoporosis. We are then exposed to a high risk of fractures and bone-related injuries.

Joint Stiffness and Reduced Flexibility

Lack of movement can result in joint stiffness and reduced flexibility, increasing the risks of accidents like falls, a significant concern for older adults.

Cardiovascular Health

Cardiovascular disease is a risk factor to which we are exposed if we are inactive. Stroke and heart disease can be avoided with regular physical activities because blood circulation is improved, high blood pressure is avoided, and high cholesterol is well-managed

Weight Gain and Obesity

Weight gain and obesity are the end result of living a sedentary life. Excess body weight is considered a high-risk factor for several health issues. We all know that obesity is unhealthy and that type 2 diabetes, high blood pressure, and even some types of cancer are the health conditions that will affect us if we are overweight and obese.

Metabolic Health

Physical inactivity can negatively impact metabolism, resulting in insulin resistance and an accelerated risk of type 2 diabetes. Poor metabolic health is a common feature of aging, and inactivity can aggravate these issues.

Cognitive Decline

Physical inactivity has been linked to compromised cognitive health and increased risk of age-related cognitive decline. Inactivity may contribute to a high level of risk for dementia and Alzheimer's disease to occur.

Mood and Mental Health

Physical inactivity is known to have a negative effect on our mood and mental well-being. Physical activity, on the other hand, helps decrease the risk of depression and anxiety, impacting our overall mental health and quality of life. Mood swing

Chronic Inflammation

A sedentary lifestyle is associated with chronic inflammation, a factor with many age-related diseases in adults that increases the risk of chronic conditions that contribute to premature aging.

Shortened Telomeres

As discussed in some parts of this book, cellular aging is associated with shortened telomeres, which are protective caps at the end of our chromosomes. Being physically inactive may contribute to the shortening of these caps, which could accelerate cell aging.

People of age must engage in regular physical activity to counteract the adverse effects of aging.

This means regular activity, not intermittent or on-and-off activity. A simple 30-minute brisk walk in the four corners of your subdivision can favor your well-being and, ultimately, your health. It can result in a more active, independent, and fulfilling lifestyle.

CHAPTER 3
DIET

Nutrient-rich foods provide essential vitamins, minerals, and antioxidants, reinforcing your overall health and well-being. Good dietary and healthy eating habits are critical as you age because your body's aging process is linked to various transformations, e.g., deficient intake of nutrient-rich food, compromised quality of life, and poor health conditions like the onset of several chronic diseases. Adapting to a healthy diet and well-managed nutrition is essential to maintain a good quality of life as we age.

Modern science has proven that an imbalanced diet and poor dietary patterns are some of the causes of skin aging. Dietary habits refer to your choices of food and drink. Imbalanced or incomplete dietary regimens may lead to diseases and aging, particularly affecting the health of your skin.

On the other hand, studies have proven that an unhealthy diet high in sugar or refined carbohydrates may cause premature aging. According to a clinical article by Dr. Andrew Weil, M. D., entitled "Does Sugar Cause Wrinkles?" sugar consumption has a sure role in the incidence of wrinkles and skin sagging.

An unhealthy diet can contribute to aging through several mechanisms:

Inflammation

Foods high in sugar, unhealthy fats, and processed ingredients can promote inflammation in the body. Persistent inflammation is associated with accelerated aging processes because it damages the cells and tissues over time.

Oxidative Stress

Poor dietary choices will result in an imbalance between antioxidants and free radicals in your body, leading to oxidative stress. This oxidative damage can accelerate aging by harming cells, DNA, and cellular structures.

Telomere Shortening

As discussed in several parts of this book, telomere shortening results in oxidative stress. Unhealthy diets may accelerate telomere shortening, which is connected with cell aging and the elevated risk of age-related health issues.

Glycation

Excessive sugar consumption results in glycation, a process in which sugar molecules attached to proteins, lipids, and DNA form AGE—the Advanced Glycation end product—which contributes to tissue damage, inflammation, and accelerated aging.

Impaired Mitochondrial Function

Mitochondria are the energy-producing organelles within cells. Eating highly processed foods and foods with unhealthy fats can impair mitochondria, leading to decreased energy production and increased celluloid dysfunction, which can contribute to aging.

Dysregulation of Hormones

Poor dietary choices can lead to hormonal imbalances, such as elevated insulin levels due to frequent consumption of high-glycemic foods. These hormonal disruptions can negatively impact metabolism, cellular repair processes, and overall health, potentially accelerating aging.

Poor Nutrient Intake

An unhealthy diet lacking essential nutrients, vitamins, and minerals can compromise overall health and contribute to cellular dysfunction and aging. Adequate intake of antioxidants, vitamins, and minerals is vital to maintaining cellular integrity and function.

A nutritious and balanced diet supports cellular health and reduces other factors that lead to premature aging, like oxidative stress and inflammation. Making healthier dietary choices can help slow aging and promote overall well-being.

Maintaining a healthy diet is essential for several reasons:

Nutrient Intake

The nutrients in a healthy diet support various bodily functions, including metabolism, immune function, and cellular repair.

Disease Prevention

Vegetables, fruits, lean proteins, whole grains, and healthy fats help prevent chronic diseases and some types of cancer. Nutrient-dense foods contain antioxidants and phytochemicals that protect against cellular damage and inflammation, reducing the risk of disease development.

Weight Management

A diet that is appropriate in proportion and balanced in nutrients can help maintain a healthy weight. A good and balanced diet helps to cut down the danger of getting overweight and the possibility of acquiring chronic diseases, high blood pressure, type 2 diabetes, and joint pain.

Energy Status

The foods you eat provide the energy necessary for daily activities and bodily functions. A healthy diet maintains energy levels daily, averting energy crashes and fatigue.

Mental Health

Emerging research suggests that diet can influence mental health and cognitive function. Foods rich in nutrients from fish, whole grains, vegetables, and fruits are good for better mood regulation and cognitive function. Conversely, diets that contain heavily prepared preservatives, lots of sugar, and saturated fats will increase the chances of having mental health disorders such as depression and anxiety.

Digestive Health

You should also regularly incorporate high-fiber vegetables, whole grains, and fruit into your diet. Eating food high in fiber will help prevent bowel movement problems and help maintain a healthy gut microbiota. Fiber also helps reduce the risk of gastrointestinal conditions such as diverticulosis and hemorrhoids.

Longevity and Quality of Life

A healthy diet is associated with longevity, a better quality of life, and curtailing the risk of diseases. It helps promote overall well-being, and individuals live longer, healthier lives with greater vitality and independence.

A healthy diet promotes optimal health, prevents disease, and enhances overall well-being.

CHAPTER 4
SLEEP

As discussed in the previous chapter, sleep is related to premature aging, and it is appropriate to discuss it further here. Good enough rest and quality sleep are essential for your overall health and body functioning. The absence of sound, top-notch sleep is the culprit of several health issues, including cognitive decline, a weak immune system, and a high risk of chronic ailments.

As you grow older, sleep disorders are relatively common in older adults, resulting in getting less sleep than you need. Reasonably, this sleep disorder may be because of some medications that you regularly take and partnered with any underlying health issues that may have caused the sleep disorders. That is mainly because aging adults regularly take several medicines; we fondly call it "maintenance." Consequently, you sleep fewer than the usual hours and self-diagnose yourself as a "light sleeper."

Additionally, you always wake up frequently in the middle of the night, especially those of you with kidney and prostate problems, to answer the call of Mother Nature. Aging adults usually complain of waking up very early in the morning and complain of not being able to get back to sleep, resulting in less and less precious rest hours. You often get up from bed tired and sleepy, wearing heavy twin-eye bags, scowling morning looks, in a cranky mood at times, and looking old. Sounds familiar?

Good quality of sleep is crucial for your health and well-being and, of course, for glowing, healthy skin. Lack of sleep adversely affects the skin, which is one of your vital organs.

Chronically deprived sleep can lead to premature aging in several ways:

Decreased Skin Repair

During sleep, your body undergoes various repair processes, including skin cell regeneration and collagen production. Sleep deprivation can disrupt these processes, resulting in a slowdown in the repair and regeneration of your skin, which contributes to the appearance of fine lines and even well-defined wrinkles.

Impaired Skin Barrier Function

Adequate sleep is necessary for maintaining the integrity of your skin's barrier function, which helps protect against environmental stressors, pollutants, and UV radiation. Poor sleep can compromise this barrier function, making your skin more susceptible to damage and premature aging.

Elevated Cortisol Levels

Deprived sleep leads to elevated levels of cortisol, your stress hormone. Chronic cortisol elevation can break down collagen in your skin, leading to decreased elasticity and firmness, which are characteristic signs of aging.

Increased Free Radical Damage

During sleep, your body undergoes antioxidant processes that help neutralize harmful free radicals. Deprived sleep can interrupt the antioxidant process, leading to accelerated free radical damage and oxidative stress, resulting in the premature aging of your skin.

Dark Circles and Puffiness

Chronic sleep deprivation can lead to dark circles and puffiness under your eyes, giving the illusion of aging and a tired-looking appearance.

Quality and sufficient sleep help maintain healthy, glowing skin and prevent premature aging. A good sleeping schedule creates a relaxing bedtime routine and ensures a comfortable sleep environment, which can help support overall skin health and youthful appearance.

CHAPTER 5
SOCIAL CONNECTIONS

Maintaining social relationships is associated with a positive effect against premature aging. Social connections contribute to emotional well-being, provide a support system, and may even have protective effects on your health and premature aging.

Cultivate social connections with friends, close relatives, and other trusted people in your circle. These connections may contribute to your mental well-being and emotional balance.

Do not isolate yourself. As the saying goes, "No one is an island." Explore ways to reduce or ease the harmful effects of stress by getting support from your trusted friends and relatives.

Have a confidante with whom you can share your problems. But be careful whom you choose. Instead of helping you, it might worsen your problem.

Join a group with like-minded members to whom you can relate. You will feel a sense of belongingness, acceptance, and inspiration. Look for a support system group that will help you in some way.

The lack of social connection can contribute to looking older for several reasons:

Psychological Impact

Social isolation can lead to feelings of loneliness, sadness, and depression, which can manifest physically. Persistent feelings of negative thoughts and emotions can trigger the acceleration of aging through visible signs of wrinkles, dull skin, and tiredness.

Lifestyle Factors

Social interactions often involve physical activities, laughter, and engagement, all of which contribute to overall health and vitality. Without regular social connections, however, this may lead to a more sedentary lifestyle, which can lead to weight gain, decreased muscle tone, and a lack of energy—all factors that can make you appear older.

Mental Stimulation

Socializing typically involves conversations, sharing experiences, and learning from others, which may help stimulate your brain and maintain cognitive function. Without mental stimulation, cognitive decline may occur more rapidly, impacting memory, attention, and decision-making abilities and making you appear older than your age.

Social Support

Strong social connections provide emotional support, encouragement, and a sense of belonging. This support network can help you cope with stress, adversity, and life challenges, positively impacting your physical health and appearance. Without social support, you may experience higher levels of stress and a diminished ability to cope, which can manifest in your physical appearance.

Social Interaction

Social interactions often involve grooming, dressing up, and caring for your appearance. When you lack social connections, you may be less motivated to engage in self-care practices, which may decrease personal grooming habits and overall appearance.

In summary, the lack of social connection can make you look older due to the psychological impact, lifestyle factors, reduced mental stimulation, lack of social support, and diminished social interaction that often accompany social isolation. You must maintain meaningful social connections to promote your mental and physical well-being.

CHAPTER 6

SMOKING AND ALCOHOL CONSUMPTION

Excessive smoking and alcohol consumption are also blamed as causes for accelerated aging and increased risk of other chronic diseases.

They always say, "Drink, but never get drunk." Drinking and drunkenness are related to each other, but one flip makes these two things in some other ways different. Drinking moderately, or what they classically call "social drinking," is different from drinking too much alcohol so that you become drunk or clinically considered alcohol intoxicated. Once you get drunk, you tend to forget your social graces and become aggressive, unrestrained, uncoordinated, incomprehensible, and uncontrolled.

What has drinking and drunkenness to do with aging? Alcohol consumption can, in some ways, affect vital organs and make them age faster and prematurely. Heavy drinkers are more prone to getting sick with cirrhosis (damaged liver), and even moderate drinkers can have issues like fatty liver illnesses, too. Since alcohol depletes the levels of vitamins in your body, especially Vitamin A, your skin's collagen level plummets. As a result, your skin may lose elasticity and become wrinkled. Alcohol may dehydrate your skin, cause inflammation, and manifest in your skin as bloating, puffiness, redness, premature aging, and, ultimately, wrinkles. This is the reason why when drunk, you seem to get thirsty because your body is dehydrated, caused by alcohol consumption.

Giving up smoking and minimizing alcohol intake can have a positive effect on your health and life's longevity.

In some remote society, drinking and getting drunk associated with excessive smoking is the normal conduct of society, and even womanizing, fathering one or two children from out of wedlock and even from different women is a symbol of masculinity. If you don't drink, smoke, and womanize, you are not man enough, and you will fall short of the expectations of society. So, the tendencies of the members of that "society" cater to the needs and norms of society — smoke, drink, and womanize. As a result, men look older than their age.

Drinking too much alcohol, combined with excessive smoking, can dehydrate and damage your skin in a matter of time, as discussed above, giving way to signs of premature aging. Clinical experiments have shown that smoking has something to do with external aging, drying up your skin, most especially on the skin of your face.

Further studies showed that smoking and heavy drinking accelerate with time the onset of aging of your facial skin. This must be the reason why a friend or a relative who excessively smokes and heavily drinks is even addicted to prohibited drugs and has a tired, mature, and haggard look. In a "macho-cultured" society, this is usually the norm of conduct. Being "macho" means a heavy drinker, smoker, and a haggard-looking character. Does that sound familiar?

Smoking and excessive drinking can both contribute to premature aging in various ways:

Oxidative Stress

Both smoking and excessive alcohol consumption may swell up the production of free radicals in your body, which stir up oxidative stress. Your cells and tissues are highly affected by reactive molecules called free radicals, including those responsible for maintaining youthful skin and overall health.

Collagen Breakdown

Smoking and heavy drinking can accelerate collagen breakdown. Collagen is a protein that supports your skin. If compromised, it will lead to wrinkles, sagging skin, and a dull complexion, giving the appearance of old age.

Dehydration

Alcohol is a powerful diuretic that increases urination and eventually leads to dehydration. Chronic dehydration can contribute to dry, flaky skin, making wrinkles and fine lines more noticeable on the face.

Inflammation

Both smoking and excessive alcohol intake can trigger inflammation in your bodies. Recurring or persistent inflammation is associated with several age-related illnesses and can contribute to skin damage and premature aging.

Nutrient Depletion

Smoking and heavy drinking can deplete any organic elements essential for average growth, especially the nutritional requirements of your body. These organic elements, vitamins, and minerals, such as vitamins C and E, profoundly affect maintaining healthy skin. Nutrient deficiencies can impair your body's ability to repair and regenerate cells, accelerating the aging process.

Poor Sleep Quality

Your sleep is adversely affected by consuming alcohol excessively and smoking heavily, which will lead to poor sleeping patterns and quality. Deprivation of adequate rest through sleep has always been connected with accelerated aging and increased risk of various health problems.

Increased Risk of Chronic Diseases

Smoking and drinking are always connected to an intensified risk of having chronic illnesses like liver and heart ailments and, most popularly, the Big C (cancer), which all can cause an overall decline in health and eventually old-looking skin, even worse – untimely death.

In summary, smoking and excessive drinking can accelerate your aging process through a combination of oxidative stress, collagen breakdown, dehydration, inflammation, nutrient depletion, compromised quality of sleep, and increased risk of chronic diseases. Moderating or avoiding these habits can mitigate slowing down your body's aging process and help sustain healthier, more youthful-looking skin and overall well-being.

CHAPTER 7
EXPOSURE TO ULTRAVIOLET RAYS

Your skin is considered the biggest and the widest, most expansive organ of your body and the only one most exposed to outside elements, unlike any other inner organs protected inside your body. Accordingly, an adult carries an estimated 8 pounds of skin and an area of 22 square feet on your entire body that you expose daily to all kinds of elements. You can imagine the massive exposure of your skin to outside elements. Besides, your skin is one of the many bodily features others can see or notice in you. People will noticeably observe how your skin looks, its tone, color, texture, and the like. It is the impression-getter of your personality. You are sometimes judged by the way how your skin looks. They said they can tell your societal status by the color, texture, and tone of your skin.

Your skin is one of the organs people see in their naked eyes. While the skin is the largest organ most exposed to the external environment and the only organ visible to the naked eye, it is not entirely accurate to say that it is the only organ exposed to the elements. Several other organs are also exposed to some extent but are typically protected within the body.

While your skin is unique in its direct exposure to external elements, your environment indirectly affects other organs. Your skin serves as a protective covering that shields your internal organs from physical damage and protects you from pathogens and dehydration. Your skin also plays a very important role in regulating body temperature and, of course, your sensory sensitivity.

The visibility of the skin makes it a valuable indicator of overall health, and changes in skin appearance, color and or conditions can sometimes reflect underlying internal issues. However, it is important to recognize that your body's various organs work together as a complex system; each organ has its own vital role in maintaining overall health and functionality.

To protect this valuable outside organ from exposure to harsh elements, it is highly recommended that you use sunscreen to protect your skin from the harmful effects of the ultraviolet rays emanating from the sun. It cannot be emphasized much how important and substantial a skin protection program you may have in life, but using sunscreen regularly is a must. It is a non-negotiable aspect when it comes to skincare protection. Always use sunscreen to protect your skin from being damaged by the ravaging effect of the ultraviolet rays that will cause wrinkles and other indications of premature aging. Your skin is like a fresh green leaf that dries up and crumples like a peanut brittle if exposed to the ravaging heat of the sun. Sometimes, skincare is usually taken for granted as you grow older. You consistently disregard this and go on with life unprotected. Your conservative approach is usually not to take care of your skin because you are old already. But still, skincare is a never-ending routine as part of your hygiene and personal approach to maintaining good health.

Over time, regular use of sunscreen prevents your skin from getting wrinkles and premature aging, which is a good protection from continuous exposure to ultraviolet rays that can cause the breakdown of the elastic connective tissue of your skin, called elastin. It also causes damage to the main structural protein of your body, the extracellular matrix of connective tissues called collagen, found in your skin cells. Once exposed to the UV rays, these will prematurely break down and may cause wrinkles, sun spots, discoloration, and a sun-worn look on your face and skin.

It is even believed that while cooking and staying indoors, you are still exposed to the harmful effects of heat rays. Staying indoors may seem safe and harmless, but you are still exposed to risky elements, so it is advisable to use sunscreen regularly, even indoors. You can avoid the risk of various skin cancers using high-grade sunscreen. Sunscreen protects you from damaging UV exposure, which means your skin is protected from getting burned and reduces the risk of skin cancer. If used consistently on a daily basis, sunscreen has a proven and significant effect of lowering the risk of developing cancerous cells, as UV radiation has been considered the top contributing element in causing skin cancer.

As previously discussed, using sunscreen is non-negotiable. It is a must that any sunscreen is acceptable but should give broad-spectrum protection against the following UVs:

UVA (Ultraviolet A)—This is the longest-wavelength UV ray and the most common. It is also the most dangerous ray because it can penetrate the skin down to the middle layer and is the most common cause of skin aging and wrinkling.

UVB (Ultraviolet B) has a shorter wavelength, affecting your skin at the top layer. This light is the leading cause of skin reddening and burning. It tends to damage the skin's top layers and is strongly linked to cancer because it damages the skin's DNA.

UVC (Ultraviolet C) - The ozone layer is stopping these rays, so exposure to humans is from artificial sources such as lasers and welding torches

Also, it is always recommended to wear protective clothing, such as wide-brimmed hats, long-sleeved apparel, and sunglasses, when outside to avoid exposure to the sun.

Using sunscreen is for everyone. Men, women, and children over six months old should use sunscreen daily. People who get a tan quickly and those who don't must still use sunscreen. Remember, your skin is damaged by exposure to the sun and other compromising elements over your lifetime, so your skin must be protected from this harmful radiation. Without sunscreen, your skin will be damaged by various degrees of burn by the sun and will age prematurely, which is called "photoaging." A condition called sun-damaged skin.

CHAPTER 8
COGNITIVE STIMULATION

Non-mental activity is also listed as one of the causes of aging. Involve yourself in stimulating mental activities such as reading, learning new skills like cooking and baking, writing a book, composing a song, writing a love story, writing a poem, writing inspirational quotes based on experience, etc. These activities will help prevent cognitive decline related to aging.

Cognitive activities are mental tasks that require attention, focus, and concentration. Despite age, your brain's development needs cognitive stimulation to promote its growth in your mental proficiencies. These tasks can improve creativity while encouraging the exploration of your mind's capabilities. These activities often involve problem-solving to help you understand how to use logic, process information, and make decisions. Cognitive stimulation helps to improve your memory, span of attention, and response to stimuli.

Learn something new because learning is a never-ending, lifelong process. Stimulate your brain, for it has been scientifically proven that it deteriorates if you do not use your brain cells.

Lack of social connections significantly affects your overall health, possibly contributing to premature aging. The following are the several ways that affect your physical and mental health that have the potential to contribute to premature aging:

Increased Stress

Being lonely and socially isolated are closely linked to higher levels of chronic stress related to premature aging. This stress has an accelerated effect by affecting your body cells, particularly the telomeres, which are shortened to cause cellular aging and an increased risk of age-related diseases.

Poor Mental Health

Social isolation can give way to conscious feelings of stress that can impact your overall well-being. A mentally depressed individual contributes to a cognitive decline and accelerated aging.

Unhealthy Behaviors

Lack of social connections may result in unhealthy management of overeating, substance abuse, and a sedentary lifestyle that may lead to more health issues. These behaviors can contribute to conditions such as overweight, diabetes, and heart disease, which if inflicted, are all associated with premature aging.

Reduced Immunity

Isolated socially can weaken your immune system. Loneliness and social isolation have been shown to increase inflammation in your body, which is a critical factor in many age-related diseases such as arthritis, cardiovascular disease, and Alzheimer's disease.

Limited Cognitive Stimulation

Social interaction provides cognitive stimulation that is important for brain health. Engaging in conversations, debates, and social activities challenges the brain and helps maintain cognitive function. Without these stimuli, cognitive abilities may decline rapidly, contributing to premature aging.

Lack of Emotional Support

A strong social network can provide emotional support during difficult times and help you cope with stress. Without this support system, individuals may experience higher levels of chronic stress, which can accelerate the aging process.

Maintaining strong social connections is essential for physical and mental well-being, and a lack of social connections can contribute to premature aging.

CHAPTER 9
REGULAR MEDICAL CHECK-UPS

Remember the idiomatic expression, quote: "An ounce of prevention is worth a pound of cure." End quote. If possible, have a regular medical check-up and blood screening, probably once a year or every six months. These are vital in preventative measures and early detection of would-be ailments that could have been prevented. Monitoring and addressing health concerns can promptly contribute to your overall well-being.

Regular medical check-ups are essential for all ages, especially for aging adults. At this time, your body will start to experience health issues and begin to wear out. Medical check-ups can be vital in identifying potential health concerns before they become serious health problems. Early detection of illnesses can lead to earlier treatment, which could help you contain the seriousness of the purported diseases.

Having a regular medical check-up is essential to keep up a healthy lifestyle, and it will help prevent serious medical issues by early detection, which can help us prevent or manage age-related conditions.

However, if you are to forego regular medical check-ups, the following factors could contribute to accelerated aging or increased health risks:

Undiagnosed Health Conditions

Regular medical check-ups allow healthcare professionals to screen you for and diagnose health conditions early, including chronic diseases like hypertension, diabetes, and cancer. Without early detection and treatment, these conditions can progress, leading to complications that impact your overall health and accelerate aging.

Uncheck Lifestyle Factors

Medical check-ups often include discussions about your lifestyle, including diet, exercise, and stress management. Neglecting these aspects of health can lead to unhealthy habits that contribute to premature aging, such as poor nutrition, sedentary behavior, and high stress levels.

Missed Preventive Measures

Medical check-ups may involve vaccinations, screenings, and preventive interventions tailored to an individual's age and risk factors. Skipping these preventative measures can leave you vulnerable to infections, complications, and the cumulative effects of untreated conditions, all of which can accelerate aging.

Medication Mis-Management

Regular medical check-ups enable healthcare providers to monitor your medications effectively, adjust dosages as needed, and help monitor adverse reactions to drugs and medication. Without proper medication management, untreated or poorly managed conditions can lead to health complications that impact overall well-being and accelerate aging.

Missed Mental Health Evaluation

Mental health screenings and discussions about your emotional well-being are often part of medical check-ups. Neglecting mental health screening can contribute to stress, anxiety, a mental condition, particularly depression, and other mental illnesses. These can affect your physical health and overall quality of life, potentially accelerating aging.

Missed Health Education and Counseling

Medical check-ups provide health education and counseling on healthy aging, disease prevention, and lifestyle modifications. Without access to this information, you may be less equipped to make informed decisions about your health, leading to behaviors that increase the risk of age-related conditions.

Regular medical check-ups are essential for maintaining health, preventing diseases, and promoting healthy aging. Neglecting these check-ups can leave you vulnerable to various health issues that can accelerate aging and reduce overall quality of life.

CHAPTER 10
DEHYDRATION

Remember the famous adage, "Water therapy?"

Adequate hydration is vital for maintaining your various bodily functions. Dehydration can affect physical and cognitive performance, especially in older individuals.

The most common factor increasing serum sodium in the body is a decreased water level. If reversed, this indicates that hydrating will slow aging and prevent chronic diseases.

It is also sad to note that as you grow older, you are more susceptible to dehydration because your thirst sensation is lessened, causing you not to drink much-needed water. As a result, your body's water and sodium balance changes, which is a natural occurrence as you age. Drinking enough water or liquid has a significant effect on lowering your risk of developing chronic diseases like Alzheimer's disease and dementia, Chronic Obstructive Pulmonary Disease (COPD), depression, heart failure, Chronic Kidney Disease (CKD), diabetes, heart disease, e.g., ischemic and coronary, arthritis, high cholesterol, and hypertension (HBP) and a lot more.

Dehydration could be a very significant risk for older adults. Your kidneys may not work well enough with age, so when you are dehydrated, this will lead to a fluid imbalance in your body. When this happens, the above-mentioned chronic illnesses will most likely occur. Remember, getting older also means you are closer to many medications like diuretics, which are known to cause dehydration.

So, the question is, "How much water should I drink?" The answer is, to be exact, eight (8) glasses of water a day. This daily intake of water will also help clean your skin thoroughly, thus helping prevent its aging. When our skin is deprived of moisture, it tends to get dry; when it is dry, like a leaf, it withers.

Keeping yourself hydrated is one of the best-kept secrets for healthier, younger-looking skin. Remember, our body mass comprises a large percentage of water; if you don't drink enough water or liquid, it will appear on your skin. Without enough water, your skin will look dull, dry, and prematurely wrinkled.

Dehydration can indeed contribute to the aging process in several ways:

Skin Health

Dehydration can lead to dryness, flakiness, and loss of skin elasticity. Over time, this can result in wrinkles, fine lines, and an overall aged appearance. When your body lacks adequate hydration, it can't maintain its natural moisture balance, leading to dull, dehydrated skin.

Cellular Damage

Water is essential for cellular functioning and maintaining proper cellular structure. When your body is dehydrated, cells can become damaged more quickly due to increased oxidative stress and a lack of nutrients being transported effectively. Damaged cells can accelerate the aging process at a cellular level.

Collagen Production

Collagen production is compromised when you are chronically dehydrated. This hinders your body's ability to produce the protein (collagen) crucial in maintaining your skin's firmness and elasticity. Reduced collagen production can result in sagging skin and the formation of wrinkles, contributing to an aging appearance.

Toxin Build-Up

Adequate hydration is necessary for flushing toxins and waste products out of your body. When dehydrated, these toxins can accumulate, leading to inflammation and damage to tissues and organs. The persistent occurrence of inflammation is closely related to various age-related conditions, including cardiovascular disease, arthritis, and neurodegenerative diseases.

Impaired Organ Function

Dehydration can impair the function of vital organs such as the kidneys, liver, and heart. These organs are responsible for detoxification, nutrient metabolism, and overall health. When they are not functioning optimally due to dehydration, aging accelerates, and the risk of age-related diseases increases.

Cognitive Decline

Dehydration also adversely affects your brain's efficacy, resulting in cognitive decline, memory, attention, and decision-making impairments. Neurodegenerative diseases such as Alzheimer's disease, which is often associated with aging, have been associated with chronic dehydration.

In summary, dehydration can contribute to aging by affecting skin health, cellular function, collagen production, toxin elimination, organ function, and cognitive health. Ensuring adequate hydration is essential for maintaining overall health and vitality and can help slow aging.

CHAPTER 11
WEIGHT MANAGEMENT

Maintaining a healthy weight through a good diet and regular exercise is a prerogative. Weight management is essential in preventing overweight conditions that may cause diabetes and cardiovascular ailments.

Keeping your weight within the standard limit is essential to healthy aging. An increased body mass index (BMI) can also increase the possibility of developing health problems. Being overweight in middle age is a very high-risk factor for many age-related chronic diseases. Eventually, it decreases life expectancy by about seven years. This is only a rough estimate if we combine the harmful effects of cardiovascular disease and cancer on an individual's life span.

Based on reliable research, it was found that an individual who cut their calorie intake slowed down the pace of aging by 2% to 3% compared to people who are on a regular diet. Losing weight improves your overall health; this helps boost your self-esteem and project a youthful radiance and appearance. Losing weight impacts your skin tones, making it more defined and elastic. Losing weight is not just about looking good but also about feeling good, young, and healthy. This is why a healthy body weight, aside from looking young, has that distinctive atmosphere of elegance.

A healthy lifestyle, including proper nutrition, regular physical activity, adequate rest and sleep, well-managed stress, and a cheerful disposition, will result in a desirable quality of life. These can have a lasting effect on your health and well-being that you will carry on until you grow much older.

Pre-mature aging and promoting overall health and longevity have something to do relatively with managing your weight.

Here are some ways in which weight management can contribute to anti-aging efforts:

Reduced Risk of Chronic Diseases

Managing a healthy weight can prevent diseases like heart disease, type 2 diabetes, high blood pressure, and certain cancers. These conditions are detrimental to your health and can accelerate the aging process.

Healthy Skin

Being overweight can cause inflammation in your body, which can manifest in the skin as pimples, wrinkles, and other signs of aging. Managing weight and eating a good diet rich in antioxidants and nutrients can promote healthy skin and slow aging.

Joint Health

Carrying excess weight puts additional force on your joints, eventually causing wear and tear. Being overweight can result in conditions such as osteoarthritis, significantly impacting mobility and quality of life as you age. Keeping your weight at a healthy level will lessen the stress on your joints and help preserve their function and structure.

Improved Cognitive Function

Weighing over the average level to the extent of being obese will expose you to a risk of cognitive decline and dementia. By managing your weight through regular exercise and a balanced diet, you can support brain health and reduce the risk of age-related cognitive impairments.

Hormonal Balance

Excess body fat can disrupt hormonal balance, leading to issues such as insulin resistance and imbalances in sex hormones. These hormonal changes can accelerate aging and increase the risk of age-related diseases. Weight management can help you restore hormonal balance and promote overall health.

Better Sleep

Overweight or obese people experience sleep disorders and poor sleep quality. Adequate sleep is essential for cellular repair, hormone regulation, and overall good health. Regulating and maintaining a healthy weight can help improve your sleep quality and support the body's natural rejuvenating processes.

Increased Longevity

A systematic clinical study concludes that healthy weight is related to a long life span. It reduces the imminent risk of chronic diseases and promotes overall health; weight management can also help extend the quality of life.

In summary, weight management is a crucial component of your anti-aging strategies. Good weight management will lower the occurrence of chronic diseases and help you promote overall healthy well-being that aids in your body's natural rejuvenation process. Maintaining a healthy weight through lifestyle modifications by exercising partnered with a well-balanced diet can help you deter the progression of aging. It will enable you to benefit from a long and healthy life.

CHAPTER 12
GENETIC INFLUENCE

In some cases, a poor lifestyle is not the only factor responsible for premature aging; your natural genes could also be the culprit. Sometimes, your genes or DNA are programmed to age your skin and body sooner than later. However, with a well-maintained, healthy lifestyle, this can be avoided or aborted.

Your genes play a significant role in your body's aging process and can influence various aspects of an individual's aging. While aging is a complex and multifaceted phenomenon, understanding the combination of genetic and environmental factors will provide you insights into why some individuals are different. Why do some mature early, and why do others do not?

Here are ways how genes affect aging:

Imbalanced Free Radicals:

- The free radicals attack your DNA, which can lead to developing cancer in your body. Regarding skin care, free radicals can attack proteins like collagen and lipids in your skin's structure, especially the defensive barrier layer.

- Free radicals are unstable atoms with only one unpaired electron. They need to be paired to be stable so that they can look for another bit to bind. Free radicals damage your human cells, cause or speed up the aging process, and even wreak havoc on the development of cancer and other diseases.

- In other words, they are molecules with an uneven number of electrons, which makes them unstable. To achieve stability, these molecules seek to acquire or donate electrons, leading to a chain reaction of electrons "stealing" from other molecules, damaging cells, proteins, and DNA of your body.

- Free radicals can be formed through various natural processes in your body, such as during metabolism or exposure to external factors like radiation, pollution, tobacco smoke, and certain chemicals. While your body has natural defenses, such as antioxidants, to neutralize free radicals, an imbalance of free radicals and antioxidants can cause or result in oxidative stress linked to various health conditions, including premature aging, cancer, cardiovascular diseases, and neurodegenerative disorders.

- Antioxidants, substances that neutralize free radicals by donating electrons without becoming destabilized, play a crucial role in maintaining your cellular health and preventing excessive oxidative damage.

- Common antioxidants include vitamins C and E, beta-carotene, and minerals like selenium. A diet full of vegetables, fruits, and other foods with antioxidant properties can help maintain a balance of free radicals and antioxidants in your body.

- However, the relationship between free radicals and health is complex, and ongoing research continues to explore their role in various physiological processes and diseases.

CHAPTER 13
SKIN CARE ROUTINE

A skincare routine can prevent premature aging because it helps in the essential steps to maintain the appearance and health aspects of your skin. Sometimes, your skin is taken for granted. You think that at this time of your life and age, you do not need to take good care of your skin. You always have reasons to say that it is just a waste of time and, most of all, money. Remember, your skin is like any organ of your body; you have to take care of it, too. You have to develop an achievable skincare routine or program like what you usually do to the other organs of your body. You are lucky that these days, skin care regimens are readily available for both men and women. It used to be that skincare was only for women. It was taboo for men decades ago, but now, all kinds of skin care products and programs are accessible and available for both men and women.

Relatively, there are products and anti-aging formulas available in the market to help you achieve a successful skincare regimen. There are also anti-aging processes that are self-help and easy to make using readily available materials. You are lucky that these days, you can easily search the internet for whatever topic you want to know, and several of those are techniques and procedures for achieving a successful skincare program.

Here's how the absence of a skincare routine can result:

Lack of Moisture

Without regular moisturization, your skin can dry up, forming fine lines, deep wrinkles, and a dull complexion. Moisturizers can help to hydrate your skin, keeping it plump and youthful-looking.

When your skin is dehydrated, you will experience symptoms of dryness, flakiness, roughness, irritation, and cracking, hence the look of aged-looking skin. Your skin has a protective gear called stratum corneum (SC), which safeguards you from dehydration - the skin's outermost layer. Its essential function is to protect your entire body from harm and potential danger from exposure to environmental toxins and pathogens that will cause adverse effects on your body. The stratum corneum is essential for healthy skin and controls the water-soluble substances called natural moisturizing factors (NMF), which are responsible for maintaining adequate moisture and many skin functions. Without the skin covering, your body's fluid will evaporate, dehydrating you. Thus, your skin needs to be protected to aid your body to perform its function adequately.

To avoid dry skin, help your skin fight against a lot of threats from outside and some from inside your body like too humid or too dry temperatures, allergens, irritants, and pollutants, exposure to ultraviolet rays, alkaline, detergents, bath soaps, steroids, harsh chemicals, and even over-exfoliation or over-washing. Believe it or not, even psychological distress can cause damage to your skin, and even genetic factors make you prone to skin conditions like atopic dermatitis and psoriasis.

Sun Damage Accumulation

As discussed in the previous chapters, without sunscreen, the harmful effect of UV rays will damage your skin, which will cause sunburn photoaging (premature aging caused by UV rays) and will also accelerate the risk of skin cancer. You need to wear them to protect you from the damaging effects of the sun. Though you need sunlight for health reasons, and you love to bask under the heat of the sun, especially during cold winter days, you need to expose yourself only during those safe hours in the morning up until 9 a.m. and 3 p.m. in the afternoon. Avoid these hours of the day, especially when it is hot sunny days because ultraviolet (UV) rays are at their highest level during this time of the day. If you are outdoors, stay protected by using sunscreen, wide-brim hats, and long-sleeved clothing.

The buildup of Impurities

Daily exposure to pollutants, dirt, and even cosmetics can clog pores and lead to dullness and uneven skin texture. A proper cleansing routine helps to remove impurities, allowing your skin to breathe and regenerate. Clean skin is always a general rule for staying away from the harmful effects of any skin-damaging elements you are exposed to in your day-to-day life.

Air pollution is an immensely harmful environmental risk to human skin. It is known to cause aging and inflammation of your skin tissues, triggering skin disorders that result in unwanted wrinkling and pigmentation.

Repeated exposure to air pollution and other pollutants over time can lead to signs of premature skin aging, like fine lines, wrinkles, and dark spots. However, the exact mechanism that causes these unwanted effects is still largely unknown.

Collagen Production is Decreased

Your skin naturally produces less collagen as you age, leading to a loss of firmness and elasticity. Certain skincare ingredients, like retinol and peptides, can stimulate collagen production, helping to maintain a youthful appearance. The market is flooded with these products, which augment the retention of collagen and help prevent premature aging if properly applied.

With age, your body starts producing less collagen. Aging also fragments collagen and makes it less distributed throughout your body. As a result of reduced collagen formation and distribution, your skin starts to show signs of aging, like fine lines and wrinkles, with dry and saggy skin.

The production of collagen can be augmented in your skin by the following methods:

1. Collagen supplements. Collagen supplements abound in online stores and even in your local health stores. There are many collagen supplements on the market. Add them to your list of mineral supplements.
2. Aloe vera. Aloe vera can be applied directly to your skin in its fresh form or as an oral supplement. Aloe vera supplements are also available in the market.

3. Ginseng. Consider using ginseng for your skin. The most effective way is through concentrated topical products like ginseng serums. Anti-aging serums containing ginseng extract help boost collagen production and enhance skin health and appearance.

4. Antioxidants. Carotenoids, such as retinol and beta-carotene, are antioxidants that can help boost collagen production. They are derivatives of Vitamin A. Topical retinoids are also available and may help protect your skin from damaging sunlight that breaks down collagen.

5. Light Therapy. Studies show that red and near-infrared light penetrates deeply and activates the fibroblast growth factors in your skin cells, generating collagen and elastin.

6. Hyaluronic Acid Treatment. This treatment works by injecting hyaluronic acid into the layer of your skin just beneath the surface. It helps to moisturize and support the normal function of the fibroblasts, the cells responsible for producing collagen and elastin.

Uneven Skin Tone

Dead cells can gather and accumulate on your skin's surface without exfoliation, causing dullness and uneven tone. Regular exfoliation can help wash away dead cells, producing smoother, brighter skin.

A brush or scrub allows you to exfoliate your skin easily without using chemically prepared products. Use a sponge daily while you shower. Start at your shoulders and work your way down to your feet. Move the sponge across your skin in short, light strokes to remove dead cells.

Products like vitamin C, niacinamide, and retinol can be bought over the counter to ease and remedy uneven skin tone. Others consider microdermabrasion and laser therapy to cure uneven skin tone. In most cases, uneven skin tone does not indicate a serious medical issue, but some people may push to correct it for personal reasons to level up their appearance and boost self-confidence.

Missed Opportunities for Treatment

Skincare routines often treat specified problems, such as discoloration, fine wrinkles, or even pimples and acne. Without these treatments, issues may worsen, leading to premature aging.

A skin-care routine aims to tune up your complexion to function at its best. It also helps to troubleshoot or target any areas you want to work on. A skin-care routine is also an opportunity to notice any changes within yourself, especially your skin, and to take preventative measures to check any problematic issues and attend to them as soon as possible. Also, your skincare needs shift as you age, and so will your products.

Get Regular Facials

Visit a Professional Skincare Specialist regularly for a deep cleansing and exfoliating procedure. This will nourish your skin and help maintain its youthful appearance. It is good to pamper yourself once in a while. You deserve it.

Having a regular facial helps strengthen your skin's protective layer, which guards against harmful elements lurking in the environment. Facial cleansing creates a consistent regimen for your skin to be in top shape when fighting off infection-causing bacteria and other damage-causing free radicals.

Sure, miracles do not happen in a day or two, but regular facials paired with a solid skincare routine can help maintain optimal, healthy skin and a youthful appearance.

How to do a simple, daily Skincare Routine

Cleanse your skin twice a day, moisturize regularly, and use products with ingredients like retinol, vitamin C, hyaluronic acid, and peptides. These products are so helpful in reducing signs of aging of your skin. A consistent skincare routine tailored to your skin type and concerns can help maintain your skin's health and youthful overall appearance over time.

Neglecting skin care can increase sensitivity and irritation, making your skin more prone to discoloration, reddish-colored spots, and other signs of aging.

CHAPTER 14
PERSONAL HYGIENE AND GROOMING

Personal hygiene and grooming play a significant role in maintaining a youthful appearance for several reasons:

Skin Care

One chapter (Chapter XIII) has been dedicated to discussing this topic elaborately. Proper hygiene practices, such as washing your face regularly with a gentle cleanser, help maintain clean, clear skin free from dead skin cells, oil, and dirt that accumulate and contribute to a dull complexion. Additionally, moisturizing your skin keeps it hydrated, soft, and elastic, preventing the appearance of fine lines and wrinkles.

Hair Care

Your hair is your crowning glory. People around you keenly observe this particular part of your body. Your hair gives you the distinctive personality and character that separate you from the rest. That being said, it is but proper to keep your hair clean and well-groomed to flaunt that aura of winsomeness. Well-kept hair has a significant impact on your overall appearance. Regular shampooing and conditioning help keep hair soft, shiny, and manageable. Trimming split ends and styling your hair can also make you look more polished and put-together, contributing to a youthful appearance.

A subjective opinion says that wearing short hair makes one look younger. However, sporting short hair is supported by the scientific fact that short hair can project a more youthful look by accentuating features of your face, highlighting your eyes and your smile, and projecting self-confidence and self-assurance. However, the primal reason to achieve a young-looking projection with short hair is by opting for a style that compliments one's facial shape, hair texture, and individual choice of fashion. With a good selection of hairstyles and techniques, men & women of all ages can adopt an age-defying aura of short hair and delight in a fresh-looking, youthful look that radiates confidence and vitality.

Oral and Dental Care

Oral hygiene is also a routine you must maintain in good and regular order, and thus, it is highly recommended that flossing and brushing your teeth after a meal is ideal. Regularly visit your dentist for an excellent oral and dental check-up to maintain healthy teeth and gums that will ensure you keep your smile bright and sunny. There is no better way to smile than having an attractive set of dentures. Regular dental check-ups keep you looking good, keep your gums healthy, and avoid tooth decay and bad breath. As you age, your teeth and gums give up signs of appearing old. There is no better appearance than a winsome smile, fresh breath, and healthy white teeth, usually associated with youthfulness and vitality.

Good oral hygiene and regular dental check-ups can prevent you from having to resort to artificial dentures. However, for some patients, wearing artificial dentures makes them look old. This is because bone resorption changes the shape of your face. The bone that once held your teeth changes, thus giving an old-looking impression.

Hands and Nail Care

Neglected nails can make you look unkempt, dirty, and old. Keeping your nails clean, trimmed, and well-maintained can complement your youthful appearance. Some people look at your nails to evaluate your personality. People sometimes judge the kind of person by looking at a person's nails. What are good looks with dirty nails?

Hand care is often overlooked in beauty routines, but it's a crucial part of maintaining a youthful appearance. Your hands, like your face, can show signs of aging, such as pigmentation, wrinkling, and loss of volume. These signs can add years to your age and affect your overall impression. By focusing on hand care, you can effectively remedy the symptoms and maintain a youthful look.

Your hands are among the first parts of your body to start showing signs of aging. They are considered the most visible indicator of age, even more so than our neck, chest, or face. This is because there is less fat on the backs of your hands compared to the rest of your body, making them susceptible to collagen and elastin loss. This can result in a thin, translucent texture that can cause veins to bulge, skin to fold into wrinkles, and dark spots to emerge - adding years of age to your hands and overall appearance. However, being aware of these early signs empowers you to take proactive steps in your skincare routine, giving you control over your aging process and boosting your confidence in maintaining a youthful appearance.

Here are some tips on how to make your hands look young:

- Protecting your hands from the sun is not just a suggestion; it's a necessity. Hand care is especially crucial when treating your hands, as the sun's harmful rays can undo all your skincare efforts. Wear gloves while cleaning, washing dishes, gardening, and other household chores.
- Moisturize, moisturize, moisturize.
- Lavish your hands with skin-whitening creams and lotions.
- In some cases, professional treatments are worth considering. Call your dermatologist to discuss other procedural options, such as cryosurgery, laser therapy, chemical peeling, and microdermabrasion.

These treatments have shown significant results in maintaining youthful-looking hands, giving you hope and reassurance about available options.

Dress, Style, and Public Projection

Dress appropriately for your age. While not directly related to aging, proper grooming also includes dressing appropriately for your age and body type. Wearing clean, well-fitting clothes that flatter your body contour can make you look younger and more confident. Please don't wear clothes just because they are in; you have to wear them, too.

It is not only how you dress that makes you attractive; it is how you carry and present yourself in public. When you enter a room or any public place like a restaurant or office, project and present yourself so that your appearance enters the room before you do. Bring yourself with an air of unquestioned self-confidence, deliver a strong impact, and make your presence in the room strong. Your presence means that no matter where you are on any particular day and place, your clothes, posture, entrance, and facial expressions deliver your first impression to the people around you.

The perfume, clothing, accessories, hairstyles, and grooming choices you make reflect your self-concept and self-image. Your self-image is what you "see" in your mental picture of yourself. What counts most is how you present and carry yourself.

In summary, personal hygiene, public bearing, and grooming contribute to a youthful appearance by promoting skin health, maintaining a well-groomed appearance, reflecting a healthy lifestyle, and fostering strong self-confidence and public bearing. Caring for your body and looking inside and out makes you look good, feel good, and feel younger.

CHAPTER 15
SELF-CARE

Self-preservation involves taking actions to protect and maintain your physical, mental, emotional, and social well-being. No one else is going to do it in a more prioritized way than yourself.

These are strategies to practice, apply, and engage with for an effective self-preservation:

Prioritize Your Health

As mentioned in the previous chapters, you are responsible for caring for yourselves, especially your health. Eat healthy food, maintain a balanced diet, stay physically active by doing regular exercise, get enough rest, and avoid harmful vices like cigarettes and excessive alcohol consumption. Visiting your primary care physician regularly for medical screening and check-ups can help prevent serious illnesses and help manage any health issues early. You know better of yourself than anybody else.

Whenever you feel something is wrong with your body, you know what you feel. You know how to decide and what to do. You are in the best position to gauge the status of your well-being health-wise, and no one else can.

Set Boundaries

Learn to set boundaries and say no to activities, commitments, or people that drain your energy or compromise your well-being. Prioritize your needs and allocate your time and resources accordingly.

Setting boundaries is a universal necessity in all relationships. It's about respecting your own needs and the needs of others. Remember, these principles are not limited to romantic relationships but extend to platonic, familial, and work-based relationships.

Every facet of your life, be it physical, sexual, emotional, mental, spiritual, financial, material, or time-related, has its limits. Therefore, it's crucial to establish effective boundaries in each of these areas for your own well-being.

One of the most crucial boundaries you can set is the one that protects your privacy. It's a powerful way to control who can access or infringe upon your personal space, and it's your constitutional right that should be respected.

Be Positive

Strictly observe positive self-talk and positive assertions to uplift your self-esteem and confidence. You are unique, capable, and deserving of all the good things in life. Affirm your strengths, accomplishments, and potential, and challenge any negative beliefs or self-limiting thoughts that hold you back. Remember, you are your biggest cheerleader and advocate.

Be with people who support your whims and caprices. Encircle yourself with people who have a positive outlook on life, too. This will elevate your self-worth and contribute to your well-being. Nurture meaningful relationships with friends, family members, and peers who respect and appreciate you. If they do not respect you, then do not waste time with their negativism.

Be reliable and consistent. Don't be that kind of friend who continually fails out. Establishing a solid and trusting relationship is showing up and doing what you say. It is like saying, "Practice what you preach," because if you are unreliable in one aspect, there is a good chance you are unreliable in other ways.

Seek Help When Needed

Feel free to reach out for help when you need it. Whether you're struggling with physical health issues, mental health concerns, or life-threatening problems, seeking support from trusted professionals, such as doctors, therapists, or counselors, can provide you with guidance and assistance.

When seeking help, it's crucial to reach out to someone who can truly understand your situation. This person should be a good listener, non-judgmental, and someone you trust. Remember, asking for help is a sign of strength, not weakness.

When asking for help, it's best to be clear and specific about your needs. Avoid being vague, as it can lead to misunderstandings or unnecessary worries. If you're unsure about the exact help you need, it's perfectly fine to express that openly.

Remember, no one is an island. It is essential to confide in someone you can trust and speak freely with. Take a moment to consider whether the person can genuinely empathize with your situation, is a good listener, and won't judge you. Reaching out for help is a powerful act of courage, not weakness. Those closest to you are eager to assist you.

To receive the help you need, keep your request simple and specific. Avoid being vague; it might make the person you ask feel uneasy or defensive. If you're unsure of what help you require, it's okay to admit that openly.

Remember, we are not meant to go through life alone.

Be Compassionate and Forgiving

Give yourself compassionate and kind treatment, especially during hard times, painful struggles, and challenges. Acknowledge your strengths and weaknesses, know where your limits are, and celebrate your triumphs and accomplishments. Forgive yourself for your failures, and practice self-care and self-preservation regularly.

Practicing compassionate forgiveness is not about condoning harmful behaviors, letting people hurt you, making excuses, or trying not to feel your real feelings. We still hold ourselves and others accountable. Forgiving yourself is not just about understanding the emotions attached to your actions and empathizing with yourself each time you make a mistake. Forgiveness is a powerful act of self-empowerment. It is one thing to say that you forgive yourself, but it's much more impactful to do it emotionally. Be a friend, and speak with kindness and compassion to yourself just like any friend would. Speaking to oneself kindly and with understanding is a powerful way to practice self-love and self-forgiveness.

Compassionate forgiveness is an act of self-care and self-preservation. Self-forgiveness has a significant effect on your own emotional well-being. It means acknowledging the emotions tied to your actions and showing empathy toward yourself whenever you make mistakes.

Forgiving others is not an act for them but an act of liberation for yourself. Forgiveness to others is not doing them a favor but for your self-preservation. By forgiving others, you are liberating yourself from the burden of resentment, not the one who offended you, because in forgiveness, there is peace, and you deserve peace. When you forgive, it is for you, not for them.

You can forgive others but never forget what has been done. Forgiving others does not mean disregarding the hurt other people have done to you. Still, it is about letting go of negative emotions and moving forward with kindness and compassion toward yourself. When you forgive, you prioritize your well-being and achieve inner peace. You hold yourself responsible for your actions but choose to forgive with kindness, compassion, and understanding.

Remember, forgiveness is not about condoning harmful behavior for letting people hurt you. It's a powerful choice to prioritize your well-being and achieve inner peace by forgiving yourself. When you forgive, you're not just moving forward with kindness and compassion but taking control of your emotional well-being. You're choosing to let go of negative emotions and move toward a more peaceful and compassionate future, so peace be upon you. You deserve it.

Be Engaged

Remain socially engaged and connected with others to prevent isolation and loneliness. To build meaningful connections with your community, participate in social activities, join clubs or organizations, volunteer, or attend community events.

According to research, cortisol levels, a stress hormone, increase when a person is lonely. Cortisol hormone can weaken cognitive performance and jeopardize your immune system, escalating the risk of inflammation, heart disease, and vascular issues.

When you feel lonely and feeling alone, make sure to take good care of yourself. Do some exercise, take a walk in the neighborhood, bask in the refreshing heat of the morning sun, eat nutritious foods, take some good rest, and get enough quality sleep; keep yourself distracted from negative emotions by getting a hobby or doing some improvement projects that you want to do but never have the chance of doing it, like repairing a broken door knob, replacing a busted bulb, or fixing a leaking pipe. These activities can lift your mood.

It is best to look for things you love to do. Take up a hobby or enroll in a class to acquire new skills that you will enjoy doing. Join a group of like-minded people and meet new acquaintances with the same interests as yours. Concentrate on creating a positive relationship with others in the group, but prioritize self-care like taking care of your mental and physical health and doing enjoyable, relaxing activities such as reading, listening to music, or learning a new skill like dancing, cooking, gardening, or even writing.

Challenge yourself to lifelong learning opportunities, explore new interests, and challenge yourself intellectually with new learning endeavors, such as the challenges of computers and cyber science. Stimulating your mind can help maintain cognitive function and overall well-being.

There is a big, wide, wide world for you to explore rather than curling up in one corner with self-pity and self-centered melodrama.

Get out and discover the world. Pick yourself up from the brokenness of your emotions, rise straight, and tell the world, "Hey, I am going to overcome all the trials and challenges, the loneliness, I am facing now, and I will be alright."

Be Grateful

Cultivate gratitude and appreciation for the blessings you have received and luxuriated in. Always look at the positive side of life, which will help promote a favorable outlook and well-being.

Gratitude is the key to a happy life and should be continuous, contagious, and practiced daily. Psychologically, gratitude is powerfully and consistently associated with happiness. It bolsters your emotional positivity, manifests good experiences, improves health, improves your capabilities to deal with adversities in life, and builds strong relationships.

Gratitude is a form of emotional purification, a soothing balm that can bring tears of joy and a sigh of relief from life's challenges. It's a powerful tool that allows you to connect with your feelings and navigate through difficult situations. Gratitude and joy are emotional values that can guide you toward a more profound well-being, offering comfort and reassurance in your journey.

When you express gratitude, your brain releases dopamine and serotonin, the two crucial neurotransmitters responsible for your emotions and make you feel good. They don't just make you feel 'good'; they have an immediate and profound impact on your mood, filling you with a sense of happiness from within. This immediate uplift in mood can pave the way for a more optimistic outlook on life.

Gratitude contributes to happiness and optimism and is associated with satisfaction in relationships and daily life. Highly grateful individuals appreciate everyday events and can cope effectively with severe and traumatic events.

Being grateful leads to accepting all that makes your lives what they are. Being grateful encompasses the willingness to expand one's attention so that one perceives more of the good news one is constantly receiving.

Being grateful highlights the good and positive aspects of life, acknowledging the good things, experiences, and people that bring joy and fulfillment. It involves a mindset of thankfulness and appreciation for the blessings, big or small that you receive every day.

Being grateful is focusing more on what you have rather than what you do not have, cultivating a sense of abundance and contentment. It's about expressing gratitude, whether to others, to the universe, or simply to yourself, for life's richness you have at hand.

Remember that self-care and preservation is a continuous process that requires attention and effort. It prioritizes physical, emotional, and mental well-being through intentional practices that nurture and replenish oneself. It encompasses activities and habits that promote health, relaxation, and inner balance, such as exercise, healthy eating, adequate sleep, mindfulness, setting boundaries, and engaging in activities that bring joy and fulfillment. Self-care and preservation are about recognizing and honoring one's needs and limitations and taking proactive steps to maintain overall wellness and resilience amidst life's challenges. It's a vital aspect of self-love and personal growth for sustaining energy, resilience, and happiness, enhancing the quality of life, and more effectively navigating life's challenges.

Pamper Yourself

Pampering yourself is not only a luxurious indulgence but also a priceless indulgence that will gratify your general well-being and personal development.

Treat yourself to pampering experiences that make you feel special and rejuvenated. Remember, you deserve this. Pampering yourself could include a spa day, massage therapy day, a luxurious bath day with essential oils, or a relaxing manicure/pedicure session day. These indulgences are not just luxuries; they are essential for your well-being, personal growth, joy, and self-gratification.

Be Mindful of the Present

Live and be present for the moment. Experience, enjoy, and take your time to savor the moment of what and how it is to be alive today, this very moment of the day, and this very moment in time.

Practice self-mindfulness in your day-to-day living by observing a present-to-moment awareness and conscious living. Take time to appreciate the small joys and beauty around you, whether it's savoring a cup of tea, enjoying a walk with nature, or simply being alive and breathing.

Practicing mindfulness, mindful of taking one day at a time, can be a luxurious self-care act.

Mindfulness Practice

Designate a specific time for your mindfulness practice. It could be in the morning to start your day or in the evening to unwind. Create a relaxing environment. Find a quiet and comfortable space where you won't be disturbed. Light candles, burn incense or play soft music to create a serene atmosphere.

Then, do a self-meditation. Bring your attention closely to your entire body. Close your eyes, thoroughly examine your whole body from head to toe, and check for any tension or discomfort. With each exhale, release any tension you're holding onto. Focus on your breathing. Pay attention to your breath as it flows in and out of your body. Concentrate on how you breathe and feel the air in and out of your nostrils and abdomen. Then, pay close attention to your body's sensations as you move and breathe mindfully.

Savor the Moment

Take the time to savor simple pleasures, such as enjoying a slice of your favorite chocolate cake or sipping a hot coffee concocted from your favorite aroma. Pay attention to the taste, texture, and smell of the coffee and cake, allowing yourself to experience the moment fully, undisturbed.

Eat slowly and savor each bite. Concentrate on the sensation of the food in your mouth and the sensation of eating. Chew slowly and enjoy the experience of nourishing your body.

Commune with Nature

Take a leisurely walk and immerse yourself in the beauty of your surroundings. Take a walk, keenly observe the smell of the grass, the incredible sounds of the crickets, the chirping of the birds, and the beautiful sights of the greenery around you. Allow yourself to be physically present in the moment. Enjoy and take time to experience the wonderful feeling of communicating with Mother Nature, the blissfulness of being in commune with her that you have rarely experienced before.

Practice Journaling

Reflect on your mindfulness. Practice by journaling about your thoughts and feelings. Write down any reflections, insights, and observations that may come up during the day. Take reasonable notice of any changes in your mood or emotion. Have a writing pad and pen handy, so when you need to write something that comes up in your mind, write it down because, in a split of seconds, those thoughts will be gone. It is your creative juices that flow in fleeting moments, capture it in writing.

Be reminded that mindfulness is being fully present in the moment without judgment. So, whatever practice you choose, approach it with openness, curiosity, and kindness toward yourself.

Set Your Goals

Set meaningful goals that align with your values, passions, and aspirations. Enumerate your big and personal goals into small steps that you can easily manage, and celebrate your progress along the way, reinforcing a sense of achievement and motivation.

Setting goals for a fulfilling life involves a mixture of introspection, planning, and action.

Think about what truly matters to you. What do you value in life? What brings you joy and fulfillment? Understand the real meaning of your core values that will lead you to set meaningful goals and objectives in life.

Set priorities in life by determining what aspect you want to focus on. Your priorities include career, relationships, health, personal growth, hobbies, etc. Prioritize these areas based on their importance to you.

Make sure your goals are S.M.A.R.T., which means they are:

S - Specific

M - Measurable

A - Achievable

R - Relevant

T - Time- Bound

Break down long-term goals. If you have big, long-term goals, break them down into smaller, manageable steps. This makes them less overwhelming and allows you to track your progress more easily.

Visualize your success. Imagine yourself achieving your goals. Visualizing success can increase motivation and help you stay focused during challenging times.

Stay flexible. Life is unpredictable, and circumstances may change. Be willing to adapt your goals as needed, but stay committed to your overarching vision.

Seek support. Share your goals with supportive friends, family members, or mentors. They can offer encouragement, accountability, and valuable advice along the way.

Take action. The most crucial step is to take action toward your goals. Break inertia by taking the first step, no matter how small. Consistent action is critical to progress.

Celebrate Milestones. Acknowledge and celebrate your achievements, no matter how small. Your achievements reinforce positive behavior and motivate you to keep moving forward.

Review and adjust your goals regularly. Periodically review your goals and progress.

Evaluate what's going on, what needs to be done, and what adjustments should be made. Make changes as necessary to stay aligned with your aspirations.

Stay Inspired. Surround yourself with inspiration. Read motivational books, listen to inspiring podcasts, observe role models, or find other motivational sources that keep you energized and enthusiastic about your goals.

It is never too late to be engaged, even at an advanced age, because there is no better way to live than to live, feel, and look young, even beyond age.

CHAPTER 16
CONCLUSION

It is important to note that these theories are not exclusive, and premature aging is a combination of all these factors, as mentioned above. Presently, research aims to deeply understand the aging process and explore potential interventions to promote healthy aging.

While it's widely understood that the above-mentioned causes can have adverse effects on your health, including mental and physical aspects of your well-being, and most especially on your looks and personal appearance, it's still very important to express in elaboration for the following objectives:

Awareness

Not everyone may be fully aware of how much the above causes can impact health. Explaining and educating people helps increase awareness and comprehension of the effects and causes of several or most illnesses.

Understanding the Mechanisms

Explaining how the above causes may affect your body at a physiological level can help you grasp why managing the causes of aging is essential for maintaining good health. Understanding the mechanisms involved, such as releasing stress hormones like cortisol and its impact on various bodily systems, can empower you to take proactive steps to manage stress effectively.

Motivational Management

Knowing the potential health consequences of the causes of premature aging can motivate you to prioritize management strategies in your daily life to control and manage precautionary measures for better results. Understanding that the causes of premature aging can contribute to conditions such as cardiovascular disease, weakened immune systems, and mental health disorders may make you more inclined to adopt stress-reducing practices.

Dispelling Misconceptions

There may be misconceptions about the causes and effects of premature aging. Clear explanations backed by scientific evidence can dispel myths and ensure you have accurate information to make informed decisions about your health and well-being.

In conclusion, aging is a natural and inevitable part of life that encompasses a multitude of experiences, challenges, and opportunities. Throughout this book, you have explored the various dimensions of aging, from its physiological and psychological aspects to its societal and cultural implications. You have delved into the science behind aging, unraveling its mysteries while acknowledging its complexities.

As you reach the end of this journey, it's essential to reflect on the profound insights gained from understanding aging. You have learned that aging is not merely a decline or a loss but a dynamic journey characterized by resilience, adaptation, and growth. It's a time when you have the opportunity to cultivate wisdom, deepen your connections, and savor the richness of life's experiences.

While aging presents its share of challenges, it also offers countless possibilities for renewal and reinvention. It invites you to embrace change, cultivate self-awareness, and redefine your priorities. By nurturing your physical, emotional, and spiritual well-being, you traverse through the process with honor, dignity, and grace, embracing each stage of life with acceptance and gratitude.

Moreover, aging is not a solitary journey but a collective one, supported by your relationships, communities, and shared humanity. As you age, you honor the wisdom of those who have come before you and motivate those who will follow after you. You foster intergenerational connections, bridging the gap between young and old and fostering a culture of inclusivity, empathy, and respect.

In closing, you have approach aging with courage, curiosity, and compassion. You celebrate the richness of life's tapestry, recognizing that every wrinkle, every gray hair, and every moment of reflection is a testament to the beauty and resilience of the human spirit. May this book serve as a guiding light on your journey through the myriad landscapes of aging, empowering you to embrace the gift of life in all its stages.

Remember that age is not a limitation but a celebration—a celebration of your remarkable journey and the infinite possibilities that lie ahead.

May your passage be full of happiness, knowledge, wisdom, and endless grace be with you.

Here's to a youthful you,

LEO F. SEMACIO

PART TWO
THOUGHTS OF WISDOM

(Personal Reflection)

CHAPTER 17
FOREVER "CHOY"

Whenever my family, friends, and neighbors ask me, "You don't look like your age." Followed by, "What is your secret?" I answered them with a smile, "Secret." But honestly, deep in my heart, I owe you my secrets. I will be selfish if I don't share these "secrets" with you. This is one of the reasons why I was compelled to write this book for you.

My most regarded secret to why I "seem to look young" is maintaining peace of mind and avoiding stress. I do not allow myself to get affected too much by life's glitches and drama; I have had enough and a lot of it in my younger days. It is time to shine and live life to the fullest, sans stress. The rest will follow; what I mean by the techniques and procedures mentioned in this book are some of the things that I follow, observe, and strictly practice that help me look "young" even in my old age.

Peace is a state of mind, and I always comfort myself with this mindset. St. Thomas Aquinas said peace is not a virtue but rather an act of charity and love. In my case, it is my love of self that I gifted myself with peace. For me, peace is an inner feeling that exudes outward and inward in my being. It manifests in the humming of my heart and the hidden smile deep inside me. Peace is an unexplainable level of thought that produces a smile on my face, unknowingly and unexplainably. This is my secret of living "youthfully."

"Life is what I make it." This is my favorite quote. I always believe that things happen for a reason. My life is like a balancing scale at the tip of my fingers; if I want a kind life to be miserable, my life will be. But if I want my life to be joyful, I choose to be joyful, and I will be. I firmly believe in this kind of life's philosophy for a happier and stress-free mundane existence.

If I feel the world is against me, I cry if I may. I let my tears flow like a river, but I do not cry like crazy all day. After all is done, I take a deep breath and sigh away my tears. I get up and strive to live. I want to have a life. I pick up my broken me and patch it up back no matter how I look my tattered way. My life is worth living for. My life is for living, not for passing. My life is for going on, not for stopping by. I have a future to look forward to, and even though I am not sure what my future may bring, I am still eagerly looking forward to it in a positive way.

I cry if I will. I release all the mental and emotional anguish I have inside me by shedding it off with my tears, believing this will wipe away my sorrows and ease the burden of my hurting heart, mind, body, and soul. So, then I cry, but I don't let my emotions go so deep and profound that I may end up thinking it is the end of my day. After all is done, I wipe away my tears, get up, and smile. I tell the world that I want a life meant to be lived, achieve what is to be achieved and discover what is to be discovered. A lot of things lie ahead of me.

I always think of happy thoughts, which makes me smile absent-mindedly. I think of happy memories and embark on a déjà vu. I take a ride back in time and travel back to those days when happy memories thrived. I enjoy flashing back to the life of my happy past. It is a joy to journey back in time, and the best part is that it is for free.

I pick up a musical note and hum like a bee, go where the nectar is, and ferment a honey. I listen to my favorite music. Sing it, if I will. I sing my heart out. I never mind the tune; it will fix itself; I just sing at my own pleasure like there is no tomorrow. I believe music is life; it gives meaning and value to my emotions and, at the same time, eases the burdens of my mind and soul. I listen to my favorite songs, sing them, dance with them, beat them, swing with them, and it lightens my day. I carry a musical note and hum it the whole day like I have gone crazy. I do not care if I may.

I am here in this world on a borrowed note as a debtor. If and when is it due, and when is it my time to return this loaned life to its creditor, so be it. I know a lot of brainteasers scrambling into my mind. Can I say I have lived a life with a purpose? Have I offended someone in the past? If so, I am really sorry I did offend you. Have I lived a life to the fullest? Then, if I have lived with purpose and have fully lived it, then I thank the Rightful Owner for lending me this life to live to the fullest. My life is at the point of no return; there is no turning back; yesterday's memories are worthy of being cherished and remembered, be they happy or sad. I make peace with my past, for the past is done, and I cannot undo what is done because it is done. I let go of the "old" self to be the "new" self. I empty my cup of the "old" because I cannot fill it up with the "new" when my cup "runneth over." I always prepare and open myself for any life-changing moment, a new beginning, or a new challenge; even in old age, it is a never-ending process that I can never tell, and just be ready for what comes my way.

I commit to live in the present, for it is a prize for me to live in the present. I am thankful that I have survived and lived up to this very moment after all the challenges, heartaches, failures, successes, and struggles in the years that have passed me by. I am glad I was able to survive all those hurdles in life. I want to live and savor the present and enjoy the fleeting moment, for this moment will never be the same again, like the waters in the river that flow to the ocean and never flow back on the same river bed it has gone through. I do not worry about the future if it ever comes. I am unsure what the future may bring, for tomorrow is a mystery and a dream. I consider myself a dreamer, but I know that dreams are for dreamers only, so I do my best to achieve realities, for realities are for achieving and not just for dreaming.

I set my dreams high, so my aspirations are high. I want to be fully equipped with knowledge and wisdom to race against time, a commodity I am running out of. It is the twilight, almost sunset, of my life. Then, I will live what is left of my lifeline and take what is there to take. There is nothing left for me to do but to enjoy what is left of me to enjoy. I always say, "Live life to the fullest." Yes, I live it even if I do not have the means; it does not matter because life does not depend much on material things; though it is a means, but it is not the absolute end.

For now and for the most part of my life, these words are very important to me: LIVE, LOVE, and LAUGH.

I LIVE by the day and for the moment. I want it to be memorable for me and the people around me. Memories are bittersweet. Sometimes, they hurt, and sometimes, they make you smile for no apparent reason at all. Just remembering those happy days makes me smile, so let it be. I let down my defenses; who cares? I want to live my memories, be they bitter, sweet, or sad, but I choose to live the sweet part.

I LOVE and let love prevail over anger and hate. I let love overpower every negative karma. I just love, not counting the cost, not knowing how. I just love, not counting the hurts; just give love. I love, even if it hurts to love someone who does not give back to me in reciprocity; I don't mind; it is on them, not on me. I believe that love is pure when you love without counting the cost. I choose to give love, not knowing it will come back to me; if not, then I still choose to love.

I LAUGH, and I laugh out loud. I laugh so loud that thunder on a clear blue sky pale in comparison; who cares? It doesn't matter to me anymore. I throw the loudest laugh ever, like throwing my worries into thin air. Laugh as if it is the last laugh I will ever have. I laugh my heart out. I laugh in abandonment; who cares? It is said that "laughter is the best medicine" (*ctto), so I choose to laugh if it may heal the pain and sorrow that life brings, so be it. Life is so cruel, so it seems, but I am gifted with laughter, so I make it so loud to silence the deafening, wailing sound of pain, for pain is like the tip of an arrow: very sharp, lasting, deep, lingering, and penetrating. If laughter will ease and silence the pain, then I choose to laugh.

CHAPTER 18
THE POWER CALLED FAITH

Honestly, I'm not religious, but I still have an innate faith in an Omnipotent Power from which I draw strength, hope, and inspiration. I do not rely on my own strength because I am weak and powerless, but my faith fills in the void and gives me enormous confidence that I will overcome any obstacle that may come my way. Good and true enough, with that power called Faith, I went through a lot of impossibilities that became possibilities. At times, I ask myself, "How did I do it?"

This is the most important secret of my life, the reason why I feel and look young: I am dependent on an omnipotent power. This power gifted me the gift of peace and tenacity to survive stress. This inner power of faith provides me with spiritual joy and well-being. I feel a sense of purpose in life and the answers to my "whys"—the reason why I exist. My belief in an omnipotent being gives me direction and significance, which in turn contributes to feelings of fulfillment and happiness, thus the feeling of being "young."

This inner strength that comes from the power of faith instills hope and optimism, even in the most challenging times. This faith makes me believe that life will be in order and that there is an excellent plan at work, which can drive me to maintain a positive outlook and resilience to counter any adversities. This inner strength enables me to accept things and events that I cannot control with the serenity of acceptance and trust. Prayers and trust are two virtues that give me the feeling of utmost confidence. Prayers and trust are powerful concoctions of virtues that make impossibilities become possibilities, thus the feeling of being "young."

There is that inner peace that supports and sustains my joy, happiness, and well-being. There is that inner strength that gives me a coping mechanism in times of adversity and hard times. My faith gives me comfort and solace while I say my simple prayer to help me through life's challenges with great ease and detachment from worries, thus the feeling of being "young."

In turn, that inner strength and peace give me an ambiance of gratitude and contentment; blessings are poured upon me, and miracles happen in my everyday life like the sun rising in the morning and setting in the evening to give me a new day. The power of faith gives me an overwhelming sense of appreciation, satisfaction, and, most of all, gratitude. This power of faith is the secret of why joy and happiness manifest in my life, thus the feeling of being "young."

That inner strength guides me to live a life of values and virtues toward achieving peace of mind and the joy of giving rather than receiving. My faith gives me the power to overcome stress, anxiety, and depression, achieving a higher stratum of satisfaction and happiness. My joy, happiness, and peace of mind are the by-products of my faith and my own interpretation of faith. Though the concept of faith is complex and multifaceted, it is because faith is universal. For I believe, faith is a personal conviction and a spiritual conversion.

That Omnipotent Being backing me up in my day-to-day life gives me a high degree of trust and security, with a lofty level of assurance that He is watching, guiding, and protecting me at all times, wherever I am, whatever I do, whoever I am with, whenever I am in a compromising situation and adversary. This Omnipotent Being gives me comfort, assurance, and a sense of being protected and cared for. These powerful feelings of security provide me peace, joy, hope, and aspiration, simple secrets of keeping myself away from stress and anxiety - simple secrets of keeping myself "young and ageless." Though youthfulness comes from within, and it glows outward from my innermost being, just like peace of mind, a state of mind and a state of being, thus my feeling being "young."

With that Omnipotent Being, I feel like a trusting child, devoid of worries, anxieties, and concerns. I remember when I was a kid, I felt so secure seeing my parents and siblings around me. I was so trusting and assured that I knew nothing about worries and anxieties. I knew everything was okay, and my only worries were what games to play for the day.

Now, as a grown-up, I equip myself with trust like a trustful child again. Peace, joy, and assurance help me build a personal conviction of happiness. It was a very challenging time as I grew from childhood to adulthood; I went through a lot of trials, tribulations, and challenges like anyone else. Along the process, I was made into an entrenched human being still vulnerable to stress, anxiety, and mental anguish, but with the power called Faith, I always make it through the day.

ABOUT THE AUTHOR

Leo F. Semacio is a dreamer with a passion for all the wonderful things in life. He is committed to working as long as his mind and body allow him.

On the other side of him, you will find him singing, writing, and traveling. He is always seeking new ways to challenge himself and explore the world.

He believes in the value of life and is always inspired by what life brings. Waking up in the morning is a miracle to him. He firmly believes in karma and is a disciple of the sower; what you sow is what you reap.